'Outstanding……this is a book I'd want…………diagnosed with cancer.'

K▲II ……Honorary …………ant Oncologist at …………rsity Hospital,
*Chair of the scientific advisory board of SourceBioscience
PLC, Medical School Dean at the University of Buckingham,
and Fellow of Corpus Christi College, Cambridge*

'As a wellness coach and complementary therapist, I have worked extensively with breast cancer patients on integrated healthcare programmes, using many of the approaches in Anni's book. From a personal perspective, having gone through the same cancer journey, I would like to honour Anni's bravery and the legacy she has left behind. An integrated approach to cancer care such as this book offers opens up healing opportunities for patients no matter where the journey may lead.'

*– Laurel Alexander, wellness coach and
complementary therapist, Sussex, UK*

'This book is an indispensable guide for anyone who has, or is working with, cancer. It gives clear, balanced, and non-judgemental information on many of the key issues around cancer, helping people sift the minefield of often conflicting advice on offer, and empowering them to build their own strategies for getting through. Anni has done a tremendous service to us all in writing this book, which will be much valued and used for many years to come.'

*– Henry McGrath, Bristol Clinic of Chinese Medicine,
author of Traditional Chinese Medicine Approaches
to Cancer and Acupuncture Course Director for
the College of Naturopathic Medicine*

Anni's
CANCER COMPANION

of related interest

Traditional Chinese Medicine Approaches to Cancer
Harmony in the Face of the Tiger
Henry McGrath
ISBN 978 1 84819 013 9

Managing Stress with Qigong
Gordon Faulkner
Foreword by Carole Bridge
ISBN 978 1 84819 035 1

Anni's

CANCER COMPANION

AN A–Z
OF TREATMENTS,
THERAPIES
AND HEALING

Anni Matthews

With contributions from
Paula Marriott and Rob Stepney

General Editor: Rob Stepney

Forewords by Professor Karol Sikora and
HRH The Duchess of Gloucester

SINGING
DRAGON

LONDON AND PHILADELPHIA

First published in 2011
by Singing Dragon
an imprint of Jessica Kingsley Publishers
116 Pentonville Road
London N1 9JB, UK
and
400 Market Street, Suite 400
Philadelphia, PA 19106, USA

www.singingdragon.com

Copyright © Jan Matthews 2011
Foreword copyright © HRH The Duchess of Gloucester 2011
Foreword copyright © Karol Sikora 2011

Library of Congress Cataloging in Publication Data
A CIP catalog record for this book is available from the Library of
Congress

British Library Cataloguing in Publication Data
A CIP catalogue record for this book is available from the British Library

ISBN 978 1 84819 067 2

Printed and bound in Great Britain

me people are life enhancers – they only have to enter a room and their presence ergises and gladdens the atmosphere of any gathering.

will always think of Anni as one such person; with her warm personality and fectious laugh, her charm hid a very capable mind that, with her vigour and llpower, brought her success in the many things to which she turned her hand.

hen cancer struck, she rose above the 'why me?' question and instead responded th, 'if it is me, I am going to face it with tenacity and fight all I can by collecting ery force I can muster'. Medically, intellectually, emotionally and practically, Anni is determined to defeat this enemy that had hit her in the middle of her busy life.

atistics show that a third of us will, at some stage in our lives, have to face the onset cancer. Anni intended this thoroughly researched and friendly book to be a guide, ich would demonstrate the choices a patient faces in the confusing medical allenges ahead, for which nobody can be fully prepared. It has many eminent ntributors, not least Professor Karol Sikora of whom Anni thought so highly.

spite her formidable allies, sadly Anni's lengthy and courageous battle was not to evail. Her conviction, however, that some good should come of her predicament in e form of 'Anni's Cancer Companion', which she had so nearly completed at the ne of her death, marks her own contribution just as valid as had the prayers for her covery of her many friends and admirers been answered.

ope that many people will be helped through her advice and guidance at a very fficult time in anyone's life, and that it will have a role to play in our fight to nquer cancer.

HRH The Duchess of Gloucester

Foreword

This is a book with a difference. Anni was one of the world's great people. Delightful, charming, persuasive – she just oozed real character. She appreciated that once the cancer had spread, it was likely she would eventually succumb to her disease. But she fought it with tenacity in body, mind and spirit. I was privileged to be one of her doctors. She had many – and with great determination used our limited knowledge to help her decide which treatments, both orthodox and alternative, to pursue. Above all, she continued living her life to the full, however bad the situation. She made things normal by doing exactly what she wanted. Few would go ocean sailing whilst on fourth-line chemotherapy, but Anni did.

It was always a pleasure to see her in the clinic with her devoted husband Jan. I strongly encouraged her to put her thoughts onto paper to help others. The format of this book is unusual but, I feel, inspirational. At a time of great hope, with the emergence of new treatments and better diagnostics to personalize care, developing an understanding of the cancer–life balance has never been so important. This book is for patients, their families and all those who deal with cancer professionally. Choice and empowerment – the hallmarks of modern cancer care – require a level playing field of information. This book provides a unique insight into how one extraordinary person dealt with her disease and it offers extremely helpful guidance to those diagnosed with cancer regarding the treatments and choices available to them.

Ten million people a year in the world are diagnosed as having cancer. For many, it will be the first time they face a life-threatening illness with a high level of uncertainty about the eventual outcome. Although conventional treatments are getting better all the time, both in terms of reduced side effects and improved cure rates, integrated medicine and complementary therapies of many types have become increasingly popular with patients. Surveys have shown that in addition to their orthodox treatment up to 70% of women and 40% of men with cancer are using some form of complementary or alternative therapy. Some of these are simple and cheap – such as weekly group therapy sessions – whilst others, involving prolonged one-to-one contact with a professional, are more costly. Some complementary practitioners work in isolation and provide just a single form of treatment rather than a truly holistic service. There are many options available but little true integration around the needs of an individual person living with cancer.

There is very little research funded in this area. In 1982 the Bristol Cancer Help Centre (now Penny Brohn Cancer Care) was founded to pioneer the use of a whole range of complementary therapies. The initial idea was to provide an alternative to conventional care, but over the last two decades the centre has moved to a truly integrated approach. As a trustee, Anni was a major force in driving change as the centre moved to wonderful new accommodation just outside Bristol. The centre has now spawned various integrated cancer centres in both the UK National Health Service (NHS) and the private sectors. Two leading groups are at the Hammersmith Hospital and the Harley Street Clinic.

Both centres offer sessions of complementary therapy as part of conventional radiotherapy or chemotherapy. The aim of these hospital-based programmes is to give the patient psychological and physical support during a time of stress. This may allow patients to withstand some of the toxicities of conventional treatments, thereby enhancing their chances of survival. Integrated medicine is not used as an alternative to conventional medical care but to supplement and support it. This was very much Anni's model.

Simple integrated medicine strategies are very cost-effective. Counselling, in which the patient's fears and anxieties are explored more fully (not just in the context of the disease but as a whole person) can be tremendously helpful. Modern cancer treatment is essentially mechanistic, and a far more personal approach helps many people. Cancer support groups have been around for many years. Even in waiting areas, patients can share their fears and get relief from doing so. But a properly-run patient support group with a professional counsellor is of great help.

Treatment with radiotherapy and chemotherapy can be unpleasant and traumatic, and there is the additional worry that the disease will not be cured, or that palliation will only be obtained with damaging side effects. Relaxation in a quiet room with an experienced therapist enables patients to get through their treatment more easily. The visualization of healing images is also helpful to many patients through seeing radiation and drugs as a powerful force destroying their tumours.

Modern medicine often uses military metaphors. You wage war on a disease such as cancer, destroying it with magic bullets, guided missiles, targeted drugs, and you try to avoid collateral damage. Patients may find battle metaphors helpful, but achieving a level of acceptance is far more challenging. Integrated medicine can help with this. This book contains a wealth of information on the whole toolbox of complementary therapy: acupuncture, homeopathy, herbalism, naturopathy, meditation, visualization, relaxation, reflexology, massage, hypnotherapy. All these options (and more) are included.

Certain complementary therapies are already covered by the NHS. I believe there should be a rebalancing of funding to allow other modalities to be offered alongside orthodox care. For example, the cost of providing psychosocial support is only a fraction of that used for cancer treatments, many of which are still given in situations that patients may find isolating and stressful. Diverting resources to supportive care could provide a new holism in modern healthcare, bringing back the role of the healer in an era of technological professionalism.

Economics increasingly governs health policy, in rich and poor countries alike. Although we may sometimes find it uncomfortable to acknowledge, we ration medical care all the time, often without realizing it. When trying to understand the costs and benefits of integrated medicine, we should ask three questions. First, what is the cost of delivery? Ninety per cent of this is professional salaries, which are easy to determine within a defined environment. Second, how much benefit is obtained in terms of improved quality of life? Measuring quality of life is not an exact science, but reasonably reliable instruments are now available. Some believe, and indeed randomized controlled trials already suggest, that simple psychological interventions can also bring about a modest survival improvement in cancer patients. But so far the studies have mostly been too small for the purposes of economic analysis.

The third and perhaps most difficult question to answer is how much money effective intervention saves the medical care system, the patient and society. Medical care forms only part of the cost of cancer. Indirect costs to the sufferer include loss of earnings, travel and accommodation and the need for carers to take time off work. These are far more difficult costs to estimate and vary enormously. Can psychosocial care get patients back to work faster and more effectively? Probably so, but what does this really mean financially? The price tag for society in supporting distressed cancer patients is impossible to assess. Marital breakdown, family disintegration and mental illness in carers can all be part of this price. Estimating the reduction in overall medical care costs is a good place for future research to start.

The rise in the popularity of complementary and alternative medicines for cancer reflects in part the inability of orthodox medicine to deliver what people want – hope, in a caring environment, and a greater ability to cope with stress caused by the disease. The internet now lists over 300 million cancer sites. Healthcare professionals who act as the patient's agent – helping them make their own decisions on such complex technical matters as the benefits of different types of radio- and chemotherapy – put patients more fully in the driving seat. People respond differently to these approaches: some find the information bewildering and are not able to assimilate the options. Others are frightened and are pushed further into denial. Good integrated medicine is rapidly becoming an essential tool in cancer care: as the technical options increase, so the patient should have a greater role in their choice of care.

Anni was an inspirational leader. Her legacy in this book will help many and she would have been so very pleased to see it in its final form. Whatever the reason you are reading it, I hope it will help your search for a greater understanding of cancer. There is much that we will never fully understand about the disease. We are not simply bags of DNA but human beings. The memory of Anni's infectious laughter in the corridor as she came for chemotherapy is more than adequate proof for me.

Professor Karol Sikora
Medical Director of CancerPartnersUK

Disclaimer

Every effort has been made to ensure that the information contained in this book is correct, but it should not in any way be substituted for medical advice. Readers should always consult a qualified medical practitioner before incorporating any of the therapies mentioned in this book into their treatment plan, whether conventional, complementary or alternative. Neither the author nor the publisher takes any responsibility for any consequences of any decision made as a result of the information contained in this book.

Contents

Introduction

A female city executive was diagnosed with cancer and told she had little time left to live. She broke the news to her board of directors like this: 'The bad news is my life is in danger. The good news is I have no intention of spending what life I have left trying to learn the new high tech computer system.'

Cancer certainly focuses the mind. Now you have the opportunity to do those things that you have yearned to do. I probably achieved more in four years living with cancer than I did in the previous four decades.

I was diagnosed with breast cancer in 2002 and told I had two years at best to live if I had chemotherapy and less if I did not. In February 2003, with the aggressive form of inflammatory breast cancer, it was not expected that I would be alive in September or October of that year – a mere seven or eight months away.

I set a course for survival. I continued running a busy property development company but also took time to sail, ski, garden and climb mountains. (I've generally had masses of energy – although just occasionally I turn into a dormouse.) I believe strongly that knowledge is power. So I also started systematically searching for things that would help me – research that I present in this book. I describe (*in italics*) some of my individual experiences, but most of the information is general. I am very aware that many people with a diagnosis of cancer do not have the time to find out about all the therapies that can help them. This book is for you.

It is also for those of you who have survived the first, the second and even the third round of your fight with the disease and are determined to keep it at bay and not accept defeat. And it is for the carers, friends and relations who are supporting you all the way.

It is for doctors and nurses who suspect there is more to complementary therapy than tea and a ginger biscuit while you are having chemotherapy and who want to be better informed. Equally, it is for alternative practitioners who need to recognize and value the benefit of working alongside orthodox medicine.

And this book is for anyone who feels they might be at a high risk of getting cancer and wants to do their best to avoid it.

My immune system had been under extreme pressure from a nasty bout of some pneumonia-like virus in the April or May of 2002. May to August of 2002 were incredibly stressful months. A building project had gone wrong and I was the only person available to sort it out. Under the pressure of being on site, I started eating an unhealthy diet of fast foods, fatty chips, lots of quick pastas, and lots of ice cream. My staple tea-time snack was Marmite on toast. My diet included all the dairy, wheat and yeast products which I know put my system under serious stress. Then there was the wine in order to de-stress in the evening. And I remember walking up a main road in London and experiencing the pain of breathing in the toxic fumes. Toxicity is like a group of children victimizing the weakest link. I was setting up a perfect scenario for some form of cancer.

Cancer arises when cells become abnormal and start to multiply out of control. They are cells behaving badly. Cells are becoming abnormal all the time but in most cases are detected and destroyed by the body's immune system. Occasionally, our defences fail and a cancer results.

But Cancer Research UK estimates that the chances of surviving many common forms of the disease have doubled over the past 50 years. Great progress is being made, and the range of help available to cancer patients has never been wider. Cancer affects body, mind and spirit, and this book represents a truly integrated approach. It is my approach. But I feel strongly that it should be everybody's, and not only to cancer but to all disease. The book seeks to help you find what is right for you at the time that is right. It is your handbook, your companion, and seeks to offer you a way forward at all times.

Anni Matthews

About Anni

During her five years of living with cancer, Anni had all the orthodox treatments available, incorporating in particular the then-new breast cancer drug trastuzumab (Herceptin). She also participated in a number of important clinical trials including one of lapatinib (Tykerb/Tyverb), as well as undergoing an experimental form of vaccine treatment. Anni had three years seemingly free of cancer following chemotherapy and Herceptin, and then another nine months' good quality of life during a second remission achieved by lapatinib. Her treatment was mostly in the UK, but part of her Herceptin course was given in Miami. She generally combined these treatments with a number of complementary therapies aimed at boosting her immune system.

Throughout this period Anni fielded countless phone calls from those diagnosed with cancer, friends and friends of friends. She saw first-hand the extreme, almost irrational fear which surrounds such a diagnosis and decided to write this book as a means of answering a wide range of questions and worries in a readily accessible format. Her belief was that knowledge could bring hope, choices and empowerment – her personal credo being that where there is life, there is always hope. She had witnessed 'negative acceptance' and thought strongly that 'positive challenge' was more likely to increase the prospects of survival.

The important issue for Anni was her wish for the book to make a difference. Tirelessly dedicating herself to the task, it took three years of intensive research. She trawled through websites and read countless books and journals, as well as liaising with experts involved in ground-breaking research – many of whom are listed as contributors – and keeping up to date with the latest developments in cancer treatment. She then wove into the book her personal experience of coping with the many problems that are involved in living with cancer.

Anni still found time to act as a trustee of Penny Brohn Cancer Care (formerly Bristol Cancer Help Centre) and serve as a board member of Europa Donna, a group (mostly of patients) which shares information on breast cancer and its treatment and lobbies for greater efforts to combat the disease. She was also an active speaker and writer for women's groups, as well as several times addressing the staff of one of the major drug companies on her experience of treatment.

All this time, Anni was sustained by her religious faith, which gave her the ability to accept with equanimity whatever the outcome would be. But she combined this with the most amazing fighting spirit and was determined to live as long as she could. Eventually, though, even Anni's tenacity could no longer hold off the spread of the cancer. Concerns about a possible secondary tumour in the brain led to an MRI scan. When Anni was shown the result, there was not just one but 26 tiny tumours. She laughed and mockingly said it had to be a mistake, that there must be dust on the scanner. She also described the picture as resembling a beautiful night sky with a constellation of little stars.

A flying visit to the Dana-Farber Cancer Institute in Boston, USA (combined with a night at the festival of Baroque opera, naturally!) led to a revised course of drugs. But eventually this treatment was abandoned and the end came as summer also faded away into autumn.

In a poem written shortly before her death and read at her funeral, Anni told family and friends of their duty to celebrate and enjoy life to the full 'for I might just be watching'.

Those Who Helped Anni

Anni was helped by many cancer specialists, by friends and family, and by many practitioners of complementary medicine. Some of those involved have contributed to this book. Among them (in alphabetical order):

Elaine Bauchop was Anni's private secretary and helped with much of the research and typing of the book.

Jonathan Cohen, University of Miami Hospital, supervised Anni's treatment with Herceptin when she was in the USA.

Linda Crawford, of the Hale Clinic, was a tireless friend to Anni as well as being a therapist. She wrote the sections on Biofeedback; Brainwave Therapy; Homeopathy; and Neuro-Linguistic Programming.

Angus Dalgleish wrote the sections on the Immune System and Immunotherapy; Interleukin and Interferon; and Vaccines. He is Professor of Oncology at St George's Hospital, University of London.

Paul Ellis, Consultant in Medical Oncology at Guy's and St Thomas' Hospitals and at the London Oncology Clinic, assisted with Anni's chemotherapy.

Roger Frais, Managing Director of Cariad Technologies Ltd, assisted in Anni's hyperthermia treatment and wrote the section on Cryoablation.

Julie Friedeberger wrote the Yoga section.

Kathy Ibbetson, RGN, of the Strand Nurses Bureau, nursed Anni during the later stages of her illness.

Stephen Johnston, Professor of Breast Cancer Medicine at the Royal Marsden Hospital, London, was Anni's principal oncologist and arranged for her to take part in a number of clinical trials of new drugs. He also read and commented on a draft of the book.

Sara Lovick, Anni's younger sister, helped research and contributed material for various sections, particularly that on Exercise.

Paula Marriott, Anni's other sister, was a tireless source of support and helped her to find and research a range of treatments, particularly hyperthermia. Paula has also contributed many of the book's sections on complementary and alternative therapies and provided much of the reference material for the 'Further information' sections.

Gordon McVie, formerly Director General of Cancer Research UK, advised Anni about chemotherapy, particularly in the early stages of her illness.

Delissa Needham, executive television producer, encouraged Anni in writing this book and helped plan its format.

Marcella O'Brien, Head of Clinical Services at the London Oncology Clinic, supervised Anni's chemotherapy.

Canon Andrew Pearson was Anni's pastor and contributed the entry on Faith.

Dudley Pennell, Professor and Director of the Cardiovascular Magnetic Resonance Unit at the Royal Brompton Hospital, London, provided invaluable advice and support.

Tonia Ralls, barrister, was a dear friend and a support to Anni throughout her treatment.

Nigel Sacks was Anni's surgeon.

Adam Searle carried out the reconstruction of Anni's breast after mastectomy.

Karol Sikora, formerly Chief of the World Health Organization Cancer Program, a Professor of Cancer Medicine, Dean of the University of Buckingham School of Medicine and Medical Director of CancerPartnersUK, advised Anni on her options for treatment. He also wrote the Foreword to the book and checked the medical content.

Fidelma Spilsbury, who wrote the section on Breath and Breathing, is a reflexologist and a yoga and Reiki teacher.

Clare Vernon, formerly a Consultant Oncologist at London's Hammersmith Hospital, enabled Anni to have treatment with hyperthermia and contributed to the section on this technique.

Viscountess Windsor Clive contributed to the section on Meditation.

Jan de Vries, a specialist in complementary healthcare and nutritional remedies, advised Anni in the early stages of her illness.

A is for Acupuncture

Acupuncture is believed to have originated at least 4,000 years ago and is a key element in Traditional Chinese Medicine and culture. According to Chinese philosophy, health is a condition of balance between the opposing yet complementary forces of *yin* and *yang* within the body and is dependent on the body's motivating energy – known as *qi* – moving in a smooth and balanced way through a series of meridians or channels beneath the skin. The flow of *qi* can be disturbed or 'blocked' by many physical, mental and emotional factors. By stimulating, moving and harmonizing *qi*, an acupuncturist can trigger the body's own healing response through release of certain beneficial calming and regulating hormones and chemicals which help to restore natural balance.

Acupuncture involves the insertion of needles into specific points along the body's energy meridians or pathways, just below the surface of the skin. Unlike needles used for an injection or to take blood, they are extremely fine, and the sensation is often described as a tingling. Needles can be left in place for a second or two or for up to 20 minutes. There are about 500 acupuncture points on the body, with about 100 commonly used.

Although the essence of treatment is to restore the balance of the body as a whole, acupuncture can be specific in its application and aim to cure particular ailments. But, because it is a holistic approach, it does more than deal with the original complaint. Given that the whole body is being treated, a feeling of overall well-being, better appetite, increased energy level and greater vitality may all be additional benefits. Emotional states such as anxiety, depression and the insomnia that often results can be helped, and it is known to support and boost the immune system.

As far as cancer patients are concerned, acupuncture can be of great assistance in a variety of ways in addition to those listed above. It can help with nausea and vomiting caused by

A
B
C
D
E
F
G
H
I
J
K
L
M
N
O
P
Q
R
S
T
U
V
W
X
Y
Z

A
B
C
D
E
F
G
H
I
J
K
L
M
N
O
P
Q
R
S
T
U
V
W
X
Y
Z

chemotherapy (see 'Further information' below) and in pain management by releasing the body's natural painkillers, such as endorphins. In fact, in China, acupuncture is sometimes used during operations instead of anaesthetics to prevent pain, even in major procedures such as open-heart surgery. It may be that faith in the technique is required. But scans using a technique called PET (Positron Emission Tomography) have shown that acupuncture induces measurable changes in brain function. This corroboration of an ancient healing technique, achieved only because of advances in technology, gives hope to all who believe that our current inability to explain a particular alternative treatment scientifically does not mean that its potential efficacy should be dismissed.

Acupuncture is widely used in many cancer hospitals and clinics, where a practitioner who is specifically qualified to use acupuncture for people with cancer will treat you. Your GP surgery/family physician may also offer the treatment. For advice on finding a reputable acupuncturist, please refer to the information and links below.

TOP TIP

There is no need to fear the needles; they are hardly noticeable. However, if this is not for you, try applying pressure to the P6 acupuncture point on the wrist by wearing a Sea-Band (available from your chemist/drugstore). They are designed to alleviate travel sickness but are also effective in coping with nausea caused by chemotherapy. In 2007, a review by the Cochrane Collaboration (known for its rigour in assessing evidence) reported that applying stimulation to this acupuncture point reduced the incidence of acute vomiting in people with chemotherapy-induced nausea.

Further information
UK

The British Acupuncture Council (BAcC) has a list of over 2,000 Practitioner Members. 63 Jeddo Road, London W12 9HQ. Tel: 020 8735 0400. Email: info@acupuncture.org.uk. Website: www.acupuncture.org.uk

The **British Medical Acupuncture Society (BMAS)**, BMAS House, 3 Winnington Court, Northwich, Cheshire CW8 1AQ. Tel: 01606 786782. Website: www.medical-acupuncture.co.uk

Register of Chinese Herbal Medicine, Office 5, 1 Exeter Street, Norwich NR2 4QB. Tel: 01603 623994. Email: herbmed@rchm.co.uk. Website: www.rchm.co.uk

Penny Brohn Cancer Care's evidence-based information sheet about acupuncture: www.pennybrohncancercare.org/upload/docs/932/acupuncture.pdf

US

In the United States, acupuncture is a licensed health profession in 39 states and the District of Columbia. Most states require at least three years of training at an accredited school of acupuncture and passage of a national board certification exam administered by the National Certification Commission for Acupuncture and Oriental Medicine (NCCAOM). Most states grant the title Licensed Acupuncturist, Certified Acupuncturist, Registered Acupuncturist, or simply Acupuncturist.

If you are in a state that does not license acupuncturists, ask to see evidence that the acupuncturist has completed at least three years of training at an accredited institution. Check with your state medical board for the exact licensure title and requirements.

The following sites are helpful for locating qualified providers:

National Certification Commission for Acupuncture and Oriental Medicine: www.nccaom.org

American Association of Acupuncture and Oriental Medicine: www.aaaomonline.org

National Acupuncture and Oriental Medicine Alliance: www.acuall.org

References

'Acupressure for chemotherapy-induced nausea and vomiting: A randomized clinical trial' by S. Dibble and colleagues, *Oncology Nursing Forum* 2007, volume 34, pages 813–820.

The Acupuncture Handbook: How Acupuncture Works and How it Can Help You by Angela Hicks. Piatkus (2010).

Meridians and Acupoints, edited by Zhu Bing and Wang Hongcai. Singing Dragon (2010).

Acupuncture Therapeutics, edited by Zhu Bing and Wang Hongcai. Singing Dragon (2010).

A is for Adjuvant Therapy

Surgery often succeeds in completely removing the original or 'primary' tumour, and radiotherapy can help prevent cancer returning around that site. But cancer cells may already have been carried by the blood or lymphatic system (see 'L is for Lymphatic System') to other parts of the body where they form new colonies. The process by which cancer spreads to distant sites is called metastasis, and the secondary cancers are called metastases.

The risk of metastasis depends on a wide range of factors. These include the organ in which the cancer first arose, the size of the original tumour, whether or not it had spread to nearby lymph glands, and the molecular characteristics of the cancer cells themselves.

Large metastases can be detected by various forms of scanning. But small secondary cancers are frequently too small to see. Indeed, some may be only a fraction of an inch or less in size. To try to eliminate these 'micrometastases', doctors developed the idea of adjuvant therapy. This may involve repeated courses of chemotherapy, as with colon cancer and some breast cancers, for example.

When tumour growth is stimulated by hormones – which is the case with many breast cancers – adjuvant therapy uses drugs which block either the action of oestrogen or its production. Because the side effects of these hormonal agents are less severe than those of chemotherapy, they are taken not for months but for years. Adjuvant hormone therapy reduces the chances that a breast cancer will return by around 10%. And it reduces the risk of death from breast cancer by the same amount. But, of course, there are adverse effects, and these are discussed under the headings 'T is for Tamoxifen' and 'A is for Aromatase Inhibitors'.

Further information
UK
Cancer Research UK: www.cancerhelp.org.uk. Search for 'adjuvant therapy'.

US

The US National Cancer Institute: www.cancer.gov. Follow links to 'Fact Sheets' or search for 'adjuvant' on the homepage.

A is for Allergy

Allergies occur when the body's immune system overreacts to a substance that is normally harmless. The substance the body reacts to is known as an allergen, and among the most common allergens are tree and grass pollen, the excretions of house dust mites and skin shed by household pets. Some people also have allergic reactions to foods. The result can be anything from a runny nose or itchy eyes caused by grass pollen, to asthma, or even a potentially fatal narrowing of the airways caused by a severe reaction to peanuts.

For someone with cancer, an allergy is one more stress the body can do without. Some symptoms are well known, but other less obvious symptoms include aches and pains in the joints and muscles, depression, loss of hair, weight gain, bloating, flatulence, diarrhoea, constipation, blurred vision, and even dark circles under the eyes (although these could equally be due to late night partying!).

Some people are born with allergies. Others develop the sensitivity, possibly because of the barrage of toxins – insecticides, hormones, dyes and additives in the food chain – which we are exposed to and which put the body under stress. Specific allergies are often detected by skin prick testing in which a small amount of the suspected allergen is inserted under the skin. The doctor or nurse will then look for the formation of a characteristic itchy red weal. Food intolerance can also be detected through blood tests. Some people believe that other methods such as applied kinesiology using muscle resistance or bioenergetics are helpful. Consulting your GP/family physician is a reasonable first step. If you take the homeopathic route, having assessed the food sensitivity, the next step is a safe and gentle desensitization programme. Complex homeopathics may be prescribed to detoxify and counteract the allergen.

A

As a hayfever and asthma sufferer for years, the diagnosis of cancer and the real need to be as fit as possible to fight the disease and cope with treatment gave me the perfect excuse to go and see Linda Crawford, who finds the source of sensitivity using Bioenergetics, a system which measures electromagnetic energy in the brain. It was easy to desensitize my food sensitivity and keep away from my particular allergens. Linda's approach is to tailor a treatment regime to an individual's unique requirements and lifestyle.

TOP TIP

Do not suffer allergies in silence – they cause additional stress to the body. There are many ways of desensitizing the body, overcoming unpleasant symptoms, and regaining the body's natural balance in order to optimize healing and health.

Further information

UK

NHS (National Health Service) Choices: www.nhs.uk/livewell/Allergies

British Society for Allergy and Clinical Immunology has a list of NHS allergy clinics nationwide. Elliott House, 10–12 Allington Street, London SW1E 5EH. Tel: 020 7808 7135. Website: www.bsaci.org

Allergy UK is a medical charity offering advice and support for people with allergy, food intolerance and chemical sensitivity. Helpline: 01322 619898. Email: info@allergyuk.org. Website: www.allergyuk.org

US

American Academy of Allergy, Asthma and Immunology: www.aaaai.org

WebMD information on allergies: www.webmd.com/allergies

References

The Allergy and Asthma Reference Book by H. Morrow Brown. Harper & Row (1985).

An Alternative Approach to Allergies: The New Field of Clinical Ecology Unravels the Environmental Causes of Mental and Physical Ills by Ralph W. Moss and Theron G. Randolph. Lippincott Williams and Wilkins/Harper Perennial (1990).

Overcoming Asthma: The Complete Complementary Health Programme by Sarah Brewer in association with the Complementary Medical Association. Duncan Baird (2009).

A is for Aloe Vera

A

Aloe vera has been in medicinal use for over 6,000 years. The ancient Egyptians used it to heal battle wounds and cure infections, and early Greek writings show how they valued it for relieving blisters, burns and leg ulcers as well as bowel and stomach disorders.

A member of the lily family and native to Africa, aloe vera grows in hot climates and has fleshy, cactus-like leaves which are packed with a wealth of nutrients. These include the antioxidant vitamins A, C and E, plus a range of B vitamins including B1, B2, B3, B6 and B12 and a host of minerals such as calcium, potassium, sodium, magnesium and manganese, copper, zinc and selenium. It also contains 20 of the required 22 amino acids, the digestive enzymes lipase and protease, and mucopolysaccharides (long-chain sugars) including acemannan. Claims for the efficacy of aloe vera range from treating sunburn to constipation and include cancer. The antioxidant and vitamin contribution is unquestioned, and acemannan has shown some promising immune stimulatory properties in laboratory studies.

Whole-leaf aloe vera juice has been used in an alternative cancer treatment programme, and anti-cancer activity has been seen in animals. The claims are that it can kill parasites, yeast, bacteria and viruses, whilst promoting the growth of new healthy cells. It is said to help break down tumours and cleanse the body by helping to remove dead cells and toxic substances. The plant steroids in aloe vera can relieve inflammation and swellings and so could be effective in treating the side effects of radiation and chemotherapy.

Another possible side effect of drug treatment is constipation, and the barboloin in aloe leaves is a very effective laxative. Aloe vera is considered to have a gentle, soothing effect on internal mucous membranes and can help heal damage to the lining of the intestinal tract, before and after chemotherapy, and promote the growth of beneficial intestinal bacteria.

It is important to obtain good-quality aloe vera. The plants should be organically grown, and the juice should be cold pressed with no additives. Forever Living Products use

B
C
D
E
F
G
H
I
J
K
L
M
N
O
P
Q
R
S
T
U
V
W
X
Y
Z

100% inner gel and not the whole leaf, obviating the need for filtration, and are members of the International Aloe Science Council. Good-quality aloe vera products are widely available (see 'Further information' below).

TOP TIP

Use the gel for any radiation or hyperthermia burns or to keep your skin in good condition during treatment – it worked fantastically for me.

Further information
UK

Macmillan Cancer Support: www.macmillan.org.uk/Treatments/ Radiotherapy/Sideeffects/General

International Aloe Science Council has a list of certified aloe products worldwide bearing their seal of approval: www.iasc.org

Aloe vera products are widely available from health food shops such as **Holland and Barrett**: www.hollandandbarrett.com, **GNC**: www.gnc. co.uk, **Forever Living Products UK** Tel: 01243 527358. Website: www. foreverlivingproductsuk.co.uk, **Nature's Own**: www.natures-own.co.uk and **Cytoplan Ltd**: www.cytoplan.co.uk

Concentrated aloe vera tablets are available from **Power Health Products Ltd** Tel: 01759 302595. Email: enquiries@power-health.co.uk. Website: www.powerhealth.co.uk

US

The People's Pharmacy: www.peoplespharmacy.com/2002/06/10/aloe-vera

The **Lewis Gale Hospital** website gives A to Z information on herbs and supplements, including aloe vera. Scroll down to 'Natural and Alternative Treatments' on the main menu and click on 'Herbs and Supplements'. Then find 'Aloe vera' in the A–Z list: www.alleghanyregional.com/healthcontent. asp?page=contentselection/condensedmainindex

Memorial Sloan-Kettering Cancer Center: www.mskcc.org/mskcc/ html/69116.cfm

References

Aloe Vera by Deanne Tenney. Woodland Publishing (1997).

The Silent Healer: A Modern Study of Aloe Vera by Bill Coats and Robert Joseph Ahola. Fideli Publishing, 4th edition (2010) Kindle Edition.

A is for Alternative and Complementary Therapy

The term 'alternative therapy' requires clear explanation because there is a widespread muddle about what is 'alternative' and what is 'complementary'. Think of 'alternative therapy' as *instead of* and 'complementary' as *together with*, or *alongside*, or *supportive of* the orthodox medical approach and standard treatment. But this is in many ways a theoretical distinction. This book is full of examples of therapies that can be used either as an alternative approach or integrated as complementary to orthodox medicine.

Such therapies include herbal medicine, nutritional therapies, hormone therapies (for example, the use of natural progesterone for hot flushes caused by tamoxifen), and physical therapies such as hyperthermia. Besides, the goalposts change, and approaches that were once considered alternative can become mainstream.

Certain alternative therapies have had some bad press. Claims for cures have been based on anecdotal and hearsay evidence as opposed to the scientific proof derived from a full clinical trial. Of course, this does not mean that alternative therapies are ineffective – just that they have not been proven to work by the same standards that apply to conventional therapies. And, just like orthodox medical approaches, they cannot be expected to work for everyone.

One thing is undeniable: alternative and complementary therapists can generally spend more time with a patient than can be afforded by conventional doctors, especially those working within the National Health Service. Even if doctors recognize a patient needs reassurance (a sort of verbal cuddle), sometimes the time required is simply not there. A complementary medical practitioner is able to give support, investing time and understanding to make the patient feel valued and worthy of the care and attention required to 'get better' or at least feel better in themselves, whatever the future may hold.

It is part of our psyche that we would prefer to take a tea or tincture, or change our diet and lifestyle, rather than subject our bodies to the

A

perceived onslaught of a chemical concoction such as chemotherapy. You need to be aware of this, because (like me) you may almost make the wrong decision. It is easy to so fear the chemotherapy concoction that taking the tea or tincture seems the only option. Medical evidence is that chemotherapy can be successful – sometimes remarkably so – in a proportion of patients. People with certain types of cancer now have the option of taking drugs that are targeted specifically at tumour cells, that are tailored to the patient's individual circumstances and that produce relatively few side effects. These forms of treatment need not be as feared as were earlier forms of chemotherapy.

For many of us, alternative and orthodox therapies are not an 'either/ or' decision. We can make best use of both. If there is nothing more the orthodox medical profession can do, then I would most certainly look at all and every alternative therapy. There may come a time when a patient is unable to increase their lifetime substantially using orthodox drugs, or when those drugs have such an adverse effect on quality of life that their use is not worthwhile. The question then is whether to continue with the orthodox drug regime or seek an alternative, or to seek palliative care. The choice is always yours.

In recent years there has been an increasing use of the term 'integrated medicine' to cover the bringing together of complementary and conventional therapies in the care of individual patients. 'CAM' (complementary and alternative medicine) is an American term which covers both complementary and alternative medical therapies. The term is increasingly used in the UK and Europe. I have not seen the term CAT (complementary and alternative therapy) used at all. Until now.

CATs tend to be holistic, treating the body, mind and spirit. They include body or touch therapies such as aromatherapy and reflexology, mind/body techniques such as relaxation and visualization, and spirit healing, as might be done through serenity, Reiki or faith healing.

The complementary therapies offered alongside orthodox cancer treatment tend to be aromatherapy, reflexology, massage, homeopathy, naturopathy, herbal medicine and healing. Acupuncture and/or shiatsu may also be included, and sometimes more adventurous healing therapies are offered. Because the approach is holistic, complementary therapy often also involves help with diet and nutrition. Penny Brohn Cancer Care (formerly Bristol Cancer Help Centre) has pioneered this field (see 'P is for Penny Brohn Cancer Care').

In the UK, NICE (the National Institute for Health and Clinical Excellence) has recognized the benefit to patients of this integrated approach. But how much is available, and the form it takes, often depends on the individual NHS Trusts. There is increasing evidence that what the patient thinks influences the outcome of a drug or other treatment (see 'P is for Placebo'). The point is often made that choosing to see a highly recommended practitioner creates a positive expectation that this therapist *will* help. It is as if the body has already accepted healing even before the initial consultation. An interesting concept!

I was helped by every complementary therapy I tried. Some helped to a huge degree, and some not so notably: much depends on the therapist. One experience is particularly worth describing. I was on a clinical trial of a new drug. Even I had to admit I was suffering from side effects, although it was clear the drug was working, which is so encouraging that any side effects seem easier to tolerate. I mentioned the serious diarrhoea and resultant soreness to the homeopathic doctor at Penny Brohn Cancer Care, who recommended slippery elm powder. This cleared the problem up overnight. I continued to take it and had absolutely no further difficulties. Without the slippery elm powder, I think I would eventually have given up the trial, as did many other women. This simple little powder did the trick.

TOP TIPS

Don't be put off if your orthodox doctor scorns an alternative option you are considering. His or her main concern is likely to be wariness of 'quackery', so make sure your alternative medical advisor is fully qualified and registered with an appropriate body. Remember that the discussion should be about *your best interests as a patient*.

If it helps you, go for it. Just be careful when integrating supplements or vitamins with orthodox drugs – check with the doctors first.

Complementary and alternative therapists in your area can be found through lists supplied by the relevant professional bodies. It is essential to check the price because this can vary considerably (from £30 to £120 per hour), in my experience. It is difficult to know what will help until you try it. So beware signing up for ten sessions before trying one.

Further information
UK

Institute for Complementary and Natural Medicine, Can-Mezzanine, 32–36 Loman Street, London SE1 0EH. Tel: 020 7922 7980. Website: www.i-c-m.org.uk

British Complementary Medicine Association, PO Box 5122, Bournemouth BH8 0WG. Tel: 0845 345 5977. Website: www.bcma.co.uk

Penny Brohn Cancer Care, Chapel Pill Lane, Pill, Bristol BS20 0HH. Freephone: 0845 123 2310, 9.30 a.m. to 5 p.m. Monday to Friday. Website: www.pennybrohncancercare.org

The NHS Directory of Complementary and Alternative Practitioners: www.nhsdirectory.org

Survive Cancer (Orthomolecular Oncology) is a UK charity concerned with holistic and complementary approaches to cancer. Comprehensive list of doctors and clinics: www.canceraction.org.gg

CANCERactive is a UK charity providing information on orthodox treatment, complementary therapies and alternative treatments. Also *Integrated Cancer and Oncology News (Icon)* magazine: www.canceractive.com

US

National Center for Complementary and Alternative Medicine (NCCAM): http://nccam.nih.gov

National Cancer Institute's information on complementary and/or alternative treatments for cancer: www.cancer.gov/cancertopics/pdq/cam

Office of Cancer Complementary and Alternative Medicine (OCCAM): www.cancer.gov/cam

References

Breast Cancer Beyond Convention: The World's Foremost Authorities on Complementary and Alternative Medicine Offer Advice on Healing, edited by Mary Tagliaferri, Isaac Cohen and Debu Tripathy. James Bennett Ltd (2003).

Focus on Alternative and Complementary Therapies (FACT). A quarterly journal edited by Edzard Ernst that aims to present the evidence on complementary and alternative medicine in an analytical and impartial manner: www.pharmpress.com/fact.

Complete Guide to Complementary and Alternative Cancer Treatment Methods. American Cancer Society (2007).

The Cancer Directory by Rosy Daniels, Harper Thorsons (2005).

Trick or Treatment? Alternative Medicine on Trial by Simon Singh and Edzard Ernst Corgi Books (2009).

A is for Antioxidant Vitamins and Minerals

'Antioxidants' and 'free radicals' are frequently used terms, yet many of us do not know what they mean. Free radicals are the by-products of the process (oxidation) by which the body converts oxygen into energy. These free radicals are damaging to tissue, so the thought is that use of antioxidants may help maintain good health.

The three major antioxidant nutrients are vitamins A, C and E and the four antioxidant minerals are manganese, copper, zinc and selenium.

Antioxidant vitamins

Vitamin A (retinol) is found in oily fish, cod liver oil, liver, kidney, eggs and dairy products. Beta-carotene, though technically not a vitamin itself, is converted by the body into vitamin A. Beta-carotene is found in carrots, yellow vegetables and fruit, apricots and melon, and in dark-green leafy vegetables such as broccoli, spinach and watercress. Making sure that one's diet contains sufficient vitamin A is not going to stop a rampaging cancer. It may help prevent a precancerous condition from becoming fully malignant, but the evidence is not consistent on this point. What we do know is that a drug based on vitamin A (called All-Trans Retinoic Acid, ATRA, or tretinoin) is an effective treatment for a type of acute leukaemia, because it induces the cancerous blood cells to mature into less malignant forms.

Vitamin C is not stored in the body, so a daily supply is essential for good health. It is found in citrus fruits such as lemons, oranges and blackcurrants. Think of vitamin C as the immune-boosting vitamin: when a cold or flu threatens, I take a good dose and seem to suffer less as a result. By boosting the immune system, vitamin C might help the body's own defences kill off rogue cancer cells. Vitamin C is said to detoxify carcinogens, stimulate the production of interferon (see 'I is for Interleukin and Interferon'), and strengthen the material between cells, making it more difficult for cancer cells to spread.

Vitamin E is found in linseed oil, sunflower oil and seeds, avocados, asparagus, spinach and in some nuts such as almonds and peanuts. Vitamin E stimulates our immune response and so might help prevent cancer.

Antioxidant minerals

Manganese is important for the production of interferon, a substance in the body which acts as a defence against viral infection. Manganese is found in cereals, wholegrain, wholemeal and rye bread, brown rice, oats, nuts such as hazelnuts, almonds and chestnuts, and avocados, peas and pineapples.

Copper supports enzymes and red blood cell production and is found in shellfish such as crab and prawns, liver, some cereals, some nuts, lentils and carrots.

Zinc has a similar role to copper. The body's supply is readily depleted by smoking and alcohol. It is found in liver or offal, some shellfish such as crab and prawns, lentils and bakers' yeast.

Selenium is important for the production of the body's proteins, and for the liver and immune system. There have been claims that it increases the benefits of the antioxidant vitamins A, C and E. Selenium is found in shellfish such as crab and prawns, and garlic and liver.

That is the background. But is there evidence that taking antioxidants makes a difference?

A trial carried out in the US in the 1990s found that men who took a selenium supplement were significantly less likely than those taking a placebo tablet to develop cancers of the prostate, lung and colon. They were also less likely to die from cancer in general over the six-year period of study. The apparent protective effect was particularly strong with prostate cancer: men adding selenium to their diet had a 63% reduction in risk of developing the disease.

The trial was relatively small, involving fewer than a thousand men. But it was a striking finding, and there had been other indications that antioxidants, including vitamin E, might help prevent cancer, particularly of the prostate. So two much larger trials were carried out to try and confirm the result.

In Physicians' Health Study II, more than 14,000 doctors aged 50 or more took either a vitamin E or vitamin C supplement or placebo. To prevent bias, the group each doctor was in was chosen at random. The results of the trial were published in the *Journal of the American Medical Association* in 2009. Unfortunately (and rather contrary to what had been expected), those taking the vitamins were no more likely to avoid prostate cancer during eight years' follow-up than those taking the dummy pills. Neither vitamin E nor vitamin C lowered the risk of lung or colon cancer. And neither vitamin supplement reduced the men's overall risk of developing cancer.

The second study, called SELECT, followed 35,000 men to investigate the effect on prostate cancer risk of taking a vitamin E supplement, a selenium supplement, both supplements or neither. It was the largest randomized trial of cancer prevention ever undertaken. The results, also published in 2009, were in full agreement with those of the Physicians'

A
B
C
D
E
F
G
H
I
J
K
L
M
N
O
P
Q
R
S
T
U
V
W
X
Y
Z

Health Study: men taking the vitamins developed just as many prostate cancers over five years as men taking the dummy pills. The same was true for men taking the selenium supplement. And, again, neither the vitamins nor selenium reduced the risk of lung or colon cancer, or of cancer in general.

These studies show that taking vitamin E, vitamin C or selenium supplements does not reduce a man's risk of developing cancer. They do not show what might be the case in women, although there is recent evidence (again from an American study, called the Women's Health Initiative) that taking *multivitamin* tablets after the menopause makes no difference to risk of cancer, heart disease or stroke. The studies do not demonstrate that vitamin supplements are unhelpful in people who have already developed a cancer. And they do not show that a higher intake of antioxidant vitamins and minerals from *natural* food sources is ineffective in preventing cancer. So experts continue to recommend a balanced diet rich in fresh fruit and vegetables as a way of ensuring we obtain all the nutrients we need.

TOP TIPS

Use of any vitamin or supplement should be discussed with your cancer specialist: some may interfere with your treatment.

It is difficult to assess whether we are receiving sufficient nutrients and minerals in our diet, particularly in the light of our intensive farming techniques. So it is reasonable to take the recommended daily allowances (RDA) in capsule form. Ask your pharmacist for advice and take supplements with food to increase their absorption.

You do not have to take four separate tablets. Vitamins A, C and E are available in combination with each other and selenium. Combination with selenium may make them more effective.

Further information
UK
The Food Standards Agency: www.food.gov.uk and www.eatwell.gov.uk

The Bristol Approach to Supplements: A Guide on How to Maintain Optimal Nutrient Levels whilst Living with Cancer by Elizabeth Butler, Senior Nutritional Therapist, Penny Brohn Cancer Care. Downloadable from **Penny Brohn Cancer Care**: www.pennybrohncancercare.org/upload/docs/932/pbcc_supplement_guidelines_2010.pdf

The Bristol Approach to Healthy Eating: A Guide on How to Maintain a Healthy, Balanced Diet whilst Living with Cancer by Elizabeth Butler. Downloadable from **Penny Brohn Cancer Care:** www.pennybrohncancercare.org/upload/docs/932/pb_eating__downloadable_072010.pdf

NHS Evidence – Complementary and alternative medicine, *Causes, Risks and Prevention: Diet and Nutrition*: www.library.nhs.uk/CAM/ViewResource.aspx?resID=261465&tabID=289

US

For good information on specific vitamins visit the **Lewis Gale Hospital** website. Scroll down to 'Natural and Alternative Treatments' on the main menu, click on 'NAT index', then navigate via 'Alternative Therapies' and 'Herbs and Supplements' and select 'Nutritional Support' from the A–Z list: www.alleghanyregional.com/healthcontent.asp?page=contentselection/condensedmainindex

Memorial Sloan-Kettering Cancer Center, information on vitamin A: www.mskcc.org/mskcc/html/69410.cfm, vitamin C: www.mskcc.org/mskcc/html/69413.cfm, vitamin E: www.mskcc.org/mskcc/html/69415.cfm, selenium: www.mskcc.org/mskcc/html/69373.cfm

References

Say No to Cancer: The Drug-Free Guide to Preventing and Helping Fight Cancer by Patrick Holford and Liz Efiong. Piatkus (2010).

The Essential Guide to Vitamins, Minerals and Herbal Supplements, 2nd Edition by Dr Sarah Brewer. Right Way Edition (2009).

'Effect of selenium and vitamin E on risk of prostate and other cancers' by Scott Lippman and colleagues. *Journal of the American Medical Association* 2009, volume 301, pages 39–51.

'Multivitamin use and risk of cancer and cardiovascular disease in the Women's Health Initiative Cohorts' by Marian Neuhouser and colleagues. *Archives of Internal Medicine* 2009, volume 169, pages 294–304.

A is for Apricot Kernels

See 'L is for Laetrile'

A

A is for Aromatase Inhibitors

B
C
D
E
F
G
H
I
J
K
L
M
N
O
P
Q
R
S
T
U
V
W
X
Y
Z

Aromatase inhibitors are a group of drugs used in the treatment of breast cancer in women who have gone through the menopause. They were developed for this group of patients in the hope of being still more effective than tamoxifen (see 'T is for Tamoxifen') while avoiding some of its unwanted effects. To a large extent they seem to have succeeded – but they have of course introduced some new side effects of their own!

The three agents in use have the trade names (and generic, chemical names) of Arimidex (anastrozole), Aromasin (exemestane) and Femara (letrozole). They all work in much the same way, by blocking not the action of oestrogen but its relatively low-level production in fat tissues, the liver and skin. (In premenopausal women, the ovaries produce a great deal of oestrogen and aromatase inhibitors are ineffective.)

In women who have been through the menopause and whose breast cancer has oestrogen receptors, aromatase inhibitors are now generally preferred to tamoxifen because they lead to a larger reduction in the risk the cancer will return. There may also be a slightly larger benefit in survival – but doctors cannot be certain on this point.

For most purposes, the three drugs can be regarded as equally effective, and the nature and frequency of unwanted effects are broadly similar. Compared with tamoxifen, aromatase inhibitors are more likely to cause muscle and joint pain and osteoporosis (brittle bone disease). But they are less likely than tamoxifen to cause hot flushes, deep vein thrombosis, a stroke or cancer of the uterus. So aromatase inhibitors are safer.

The loss of bone density mentioned above, caused by having virtually no oestrogen in the body, leads to an increased risk of fracture. Bone mineral density can be measured and the problem identified by Dexascan (Dexa stands for Dual Energy X-Ray Absorbtiometry). This is an easy and painless test. Taking vitamin D supplements and calcium can help. So too can exercise.

TOP TIPS

As with most drugs, the internet provides a quick and easy way to look up the different aromatase inhibitors and their side effects before discussing them with your oncologist. Many oncologists give out information sheets on any drugs they recommend.

The tablets may cause slight nausea: it helps to take them on a full rather than an empty stomach. Fish and other oils are deemed good for any joint pain, stiffness and swelling that may occur.

In helping prevent many of the side effects, regular exercise is the key. This applies to the risk of thrombosis, to loss of bone density, to the tiredness that some people experience, and even to the slight depression – since the endorphins released by exercise raise mood. This does not have to be done in isolation on one of those wretched machines in the gym: try a dance class once a week, or swimming, or a team game such as tennis or netball. This is sociable and fun as well as keeping one in good shape.

Together with dietary supplements of vitamin D and calcium, potential problems may be kept at bay.

Warning: when taking hormone drugs do *not* use herbal preparations which might contain low doses of oestrogen or phytoestrogen. This could counteract the benefit of taking your medication – *seek professional advice.*

Further information
UK

Cancernet.co.uk: www.cancernet.co.uk

Cancer Research UK: www.cancerhelp.org.uk

US

American Cancer Society: www.cancer.org

A
B
C
D
E
F
G
H
I
J
K
L
M
N
O
P
Q
R
S
T
U
V
W
X
Y
Z

A   A is for Aromatherapy

B
C
D
E
F
G
H
I
J
K
L
M
N
O
P
Q
R
S
T
U
V
W
X
Y
Z

Aromatherapy encourages the body to heal itself by instilling a sense of well-being and of physical, emotional and mental balance. It helps to reduce anxiety and stress, and can also be mood-changing, relaxing or stimulating. Aromatherapy uses pure natural oils from flowers, fruits, herbs and trees. There are over 150 essential oils, usually concentrated, endowed with many therapeutic properties. The oils are mixed with a carrier and applied using a gentle massage technique. The carrier oil is typically almond, grapeseed or sunflower, the ratio of essential oil to carrier oil being one drop to five millilitres. As the essential oils come in different strengths and can be toxic in concentrated doses, it is best to consult an aromatherapist in the first instance.

Aromatherapy has become very popular in the last decade but is not a new therapy. It was used by the ancient Egyptians and in China in 2000 BC. Historically, healing has always been interlinked with religion and the role of plants is a common thread in religious practice. Muslims used rose attar and oud from the agar tree as an antibacterial medicine in the same way that Christians used frankincense, a known antiseptic.

The essential oils can also be used in steam inhalation or oil burners. Essential oil is dropped into a bowl of steaming water and inhaled, usually from under a towel – brilliant for clearing the head and sinuses! Drops can be put into a bath, but take care. These oils in their concentrated form can burn the skin so always add to a carrier oil first. Breathing in the vapours helps the oils enter the body where it is thought that they can bring about powerful changes to the nervous system.

TOP TIP

Buy the best natural products and beware synthetic copies on the market. Make use of any plants and herbs you may have in your garden such as lavender, rosemary and sage.

A water spray with your favourite oil can radically change the atmosphere in your 'zone' – particularly when something stressful is happening, like chemotherapy or an MRI scan.

Further information
UK
Penny Brohn Cancer Care's evidence-based information sheet about aromatherapy: www.pennybrohncancercare.org/upload/docs/932/aromatherapy.pdf

International Federation of Aromatherapists, 7B Walpole Court, Ealing Green, Ealing, London W5 5ED. Tel: 020 8567 2243. Website: www.ifaroma.org

The International Federation of Professional Aromatherapists (IFPA), 82 Ashby Road, Hinckley, Leicestershire LE10 1SN. Tel: 01455 637987. Email: admin@ifparoma.org. Website: www.ifparoma.org

The Aromatherapy Council, PO Box 6522, Desborough, Kettering, Northants NN14 2YX. Tel: 0870 7743477. Email: info@aromatherapy council.co.uk. Website: www.aromatherapycouncil.co.uk

US
National Association for Holistic Aromatherapy: www.naha.org

For a sceptical view, see **The Skeptic's Dictionary**: www.skepdic.com/aroma.html

References
The Fragrant Pharmacy: A Complete Guide to Aromatherapy and Essential Oils by Valerie Ann Worwood. Bantam Books (1991).

Aromatherapy for Healing the Spirit: A Guide to Restoring Mental and Emotional Balance Through Essential Oils by Gabriel Mojay. Gaia Books (2000).

A is for Art and Music Therapy

Penny Brohn Cancer Care (formerly Bristol Cancer Help Centre) considers art and other creative therapies an important means to transform the experience of cancer.

A study in the United States has shown that four weeks of music therapy helps patients with Alzheimer's disease to sleep better, probably because the experience increases levels of melatonin, a hormone involved in sleep regulation but also

A
B
C
D
E
F
G
H
I
J
K
L
M
N
O
P
Q
R
S
T
U
V
W
X
Y
Z

influencing the immune system. More recently, a controlled study from Montpellier in France found that music therapy led to a greater improvement in depression and anxiety in patients with dementia than participation in reading.

The use of artistic expression can help those with – or without – cancer to express themselves, to overcome inner blocks or fears and thereby find a path towards healing. Perhaps art and music serve to reconnect us with our emotions, which can be a release and helpful in coping with or recovering from illness.

For example, a person with cancer may not be aware they are suppressing anger at the diagnosis and illness. Discussions with the doctor are often controlled and rational but rarely involve how a person feels deep down. Art helps to deal with repressed anger. In art class you may draw a surreal landscape – a huge lake, which is boiling and bright red – indicative of deep anger. This is art helping to identify the problem and the first step towards dealing with it. What follows is easier understanding and compassion for how you may feel inside. It is the same with music therapy.

When you listen to music, do you find your mood changes along with it? You become relaxed with soothing music, stirred by spirited music, and can be moved to tears. I remember feeling a distinct lump in my throat at a rugby international (the only one I have attended: France v England) when the National Anthem was played. Emotion overcame the sub-zero temperatures! Music affects the emotions and/or can bring about (embarrassingly quickly in my case) an emotional state. Can this help with cancer?

A patient may choose the cymbals and crash them dramatically in a cacophony of sound as a representation of fury. For a patient to identify and accept their feelings is important. It is essential to understand that it is perfectly acceptable to own and express one's feelings without guilt, self-criticism or fear of rebuke.

Art and music are therefore tools to help you recognize issues and smooth the road to recovery. These therapies can help to achieve a greater insight and aid reflection on the diagnosis of cancer or any aspect of treatment and care.

TOP TIP

You don't have to be good at art or music. This is not about talent. It is about expressing your feelings.

Further information

UK

Penny Brohn Cancer Care's evidence-based information sheet about art therapy: www.pennybrohncancercare.org/upload/docs/932/arttherapy.pdf, and music therapy: www.pennybrohncancercare.org/upload/docs/932/musictherapy.pdf. A specialist art therapist can be found at certain cancer clinics and at Penny Brohn Cancer Care where art therapy is included in the week's course (see 'P is for Penny Brohn Cancer Care'). For those living close to Bristol, there is a group art therapy session lasting around an hour and a half.

The British Association of Art Therapists (BAAT), 24–27 White Lion Street, London N1 9PD. Tel: 020 7686 4216. Website: www.baat.org

US

American Art Therapy Association: www.arttherapy.org

American Music Therapy Association: www.musictherapy.org

References

'Music therapy increases serum melatonin levels in patients with Alzheimer's Disease' by F. Tims and colleagues. *Alternative Therapies in Health and Medicine* 1999, volume 5.

The Music Effect: Music Physiology and Clinical Applications by Daniel J. Schneck, Dorita S. Berger and George D. Patrick. Jessica Kingsley Publishers (2006).

The Artist's Way – 10th Anniversary Edition by Julia Cameron. Jeremy P. Tarcher (2007).

The Mozart Effect: Tapping the Power of Music to Heal the Body, Strengthen the Mind, and Unlock the Creative Spirit by Don Campbell. Mobius (2002).

A is for Astragalus

Astragalus (*Astragalus membranaceus* – also called milk vetch root, yellow vetch, huang-qi and bok kay) is a herb found in north-east China and Mongolia. Traditionally, the root is used in Chinese medicine as a *chi* (life force) tonic to balance the immune system and help fight viral infections, to cleanse the liver and kidneys, to improve circulation and balance blood pressure, to improve respiration and lung function, ease asthma, balance the effects of stress, improve digestion and stop and relieve cold sores. It is also said to help the healing process of burns.

Cancer patients in China are prescribed astragalus in conjunction with some chemotherapies because it contains a polysaccharide which supports the immune system and protects good cellular growth. Some chemotherapies can have an adverse effect on the production of white cells, and astragalus may stimulate natural killer cell and T-cell activity. There are claims that it can help repair damage caused by chemotherapy and radiotherapy, decreasing the toxic effect and balancing energy levels.

TOP TIP

Professional advice must be sought when combining any herbs with orthodox medicine.

Further information
UK

The Register of Chinese Herbal Medicine (RCHM), Office 5, 1 Exeter Street, Norwich NR2 4QB. Tel: 01603 623994. Email: herbmed@rchm.co.uk. Website: www.rchm.co.uk

The National Institute of Medical Herbalists (NIMH), Elm House, 54 Mary Arches Street, Exeter EX4 3BA. Tel: 01392 426022. Email: info@nigh.org.uk. Website: www.nimh.org.uk

British Herbal Medicine Association (BHMA), PO Box 583, Exeter EX1 9GX. Tel: 0845 680 1134. Email: secretary@bhma.info. Website: www.bhma.info

The Nutri Centre, Unit 3, Kendal Court, Kendal Avenue, London W3 0RU. Tel: 0845 602 6744. Email: admin@nutricentre.com. Website: www.nutricentre.com

Argyll Herbs, Unit 2, Quantock Parade, North Petherton, Somerset TA6 6TN. Tel: 0845 8630679. Website: www.argyllherbsdirect.co.uk

Shop@PennyBrohn Tel: 01275 370112. Website: www.shopatpennybrohn.com

US

National Center for Complementary and Alternative Medicine (NCCAM), NCCAM Clearinghouse, PO Box 9723, Gaithersburg MD 20898. Tel: 1 888 64 6226. Website: http://nccam.nih.gov/health/astragalus

Lewis Gale Hospital website. Scroll down to 'Natural and Alternative Treatments' on the main menu and click on 'Herbs and Supplements'. Then find 'Astragalus' in the A–Z list: www.alleghanyregional.com/healthcontent. asp?page=contentselection/condensedmainindex

Memorial Sloan-Kettering Cancer Center: www.mskcc.org/mskcc/html/69128.cfm

Nutrition Research Center: www.nutritionresearchcenter.org/healthnews/astragalus-possesses-potent-benefits, and type 'astragalus' into the search box.

References

What Really Works in Natural Health by Susan Clark. Bantam (2004).

Traditional Chinese Medicine Approaches to Cancer: Harmony in the Face of the Tiger by Henry McGrath. Singing Dragon (2009).

A is for Aura

The human aura (or personal energy field) is said to be an energy field that surrounds our physical bodies. It includes, but is not limited to, light and colour, sound, and thermal and electromagnetic energy. The strength and intensity of the auric field is thought to reflect the health of the body, mind and spirit.

Some people can see an aura coming from the energy of the body; some can feel heat or body warmth from an aura; and others report 'vibes'. How many times have you heard at a party 'I really liked her energy', 'I got bad vibes just talking to him' or 'the room lit up when he walked in'? Sometimes the language we use refers to things that we cannot explain.

I do not know whether a diagnosis of cancer increases your awareness of issues to do with energy, or whether it is simply a matter of where enquiries about the disease lead you. But I am significantly more aware of the effect that other people, sometimes close friends, have on my energy level. In the days before cancer, I did not particularly notice if I felt drained after a long telephone call about other people's problems. Now it is almost as if they had logged on to my energy, refuelled, and gone back off into orbit fighting fit. These 'leaks' or 'blips' in the auric field can be detected and repaired.

Perish the thought that any friend envies you your cancer – but it has been known. Suddenly YOU are the centre of attention. You are surrounded by everyone's love, support and caring – except for that jealous friend who is busy aiming negative thoughts in your direction, thoughts which can disrupt and chip away at your auric field.

In 1939, the Russian Semyon Kirlian discovered (or perhaps rediscovered) that electricity can cause objects to produce a discharge which forms an image on a photographic plate. The process of Kirlian photography which carries his name is said to capture the aura's individual colours, and some claim that this helps decipher the feelings and emotions of your inner being. But others suggest that such phenomena can be explained in terms of more established principles of physics.

TOP TIP

Having a focus on cancer in life could be a fun opportunity for learning about 'psychic' ways and developing your sixth sense.

Further information

UK

For courses in psychic development/healing or to see a spiritual healer, contact the **College of Psychic Studies**, 16 Queensberry Place, London, SW7 2EB. Website: www.collegeofpsychicstudies.co.uk

US

For a sceptical view see **Quackwatch**: www.quackwatch.org/01Quackery RelatedTopics/kirlian.html, or **The Skeptic's Dictionary**: www.skepdic. com/essays/energyhealing.htm

References

Stepping Stones Into the Unknown: An Inspirational Guide to Your Intuitions and Sixth Sense by Veronika Strong. DFH Publications (1997).

The Healer's Manual: A Beginner's Guide to Energy Healing by Ted Andrews. Llewellyn Publications (2007).

Anything Can Be Healed by Martin Brofman. Findhorn Press (2003).

A is for Ayurveda

A
B
C
D
E
F
G
H
I
J
K
L
M
N
O
P
Q
R
S
T
U
V
W
X
Y
Z

Ayurveda, meaning the knowledge of life or science of life, is based on ancient Indian Vedic philosophies and has been practised for over 3,000 years. The term 'Ayurvedic' is often used to describe medicine, diet, yoga, meditation and panchakarma (a form of detoxification). It is a holistic (see 'H is for Holistic') philosophy in that it treats the body as a whole and incorporates mind, body and spirit.

There may be much value in this philosophy for people affected by cancer, for carers and for those who might be at high risk of the disease, as well as everyone else who seeks a healthier lifestyle. It works on the premise that the pressures and demands of today's pace of life result in overwhelmed, exhausted, agitated and stressed people who are fundamentally imbalanced, physically, mentally and spiritually.

Following the Ayurvedic way is a more drastic lifestyle change for some than for others – but one can become quite hooked. The vocabulary is complicated. The three terms 'sattvic', 'rajasic' and 'tamasic' identify the kind of person you are and what activities, animals, foods and plants go with your personality. Most people find that they are a combination of all three, but to aim for the sattva is to tread the middle path, making simple gradual changes to lifestyle with profound effect.

One such change is, of course, diet. The tamasic diet is processed junk food, appealing to our laziness or ignorance about what we eat. Interestingly, it is also described as 'deceitful', which seems a strange word to use about food, but, on reflection, true. We assume that fast food gives us energy and protein – just that it is quick about it. But, in fact, it may be giving us too much of substances we do not really need such as saturated fats and salt, as well as colourings and preservatives. In contrast, the sattva way is to eat organically grown foods, fresh vegetables and fruits, grains, nuts, seeds, honey, salads, freshly prepared fruit juices and herbal teas, and, whilst ill or convalescing, steamed vegetables and soups.

A
B
C
D
E
F
G
H
I
J
K
L
M
N
O
P
Q
R
S
T
U
V
W
X
Y
Z

The way food is eaten is also important. This should not be done on the move, not in the car, not in an emotional state, and not whilst watching TV. This is not a way of eating designed to promote good health and well-being.

Ayurvedic medicine is part of Hindu philosophy and culture. It is becoming popular in the UK, but there are few fully qualified Ayurvedic practitioners who have completed a five-year degree course in India and an internship in an Ayurvedic hospital. So care must be taken in selecting a practitioner.

TOP TIP

The discipline involved will not suit everyone, but parts of the Ayurvedic teaching are extremely useful as tools to cope with a diagnosis of cancer and living through and with the disease.

Further information

UK

College of Ayurveda, 20 Annes Grove, Great Linford, Milton Keynes, Bucks MK14 5DR. Tel: 01908 664518. Email: info@ayurvedacollege.org. uk. Website: www.ayurvedacollege.org.uk

Shymala Ayurveda, 152 Holland Park Avenue, London W11 4UH. Tel: 020 7348 0018. Email: enquiries@shymalaayurveda.com. Website: www. shymalaayurveda.com

US

For a list of qualified practitioners of Ayurvedic medicine in your area, contact the **National Institute of Ayurvedic Medicine (NIAM)**: www. niam.com

For a sceptical view on Ayurvedic medicine see **The Skeptic's Dictionary**: www.skepdic.com/ayurvedic.html

References

The Complete Illustrated Guide to Ayurveda: The Ancient Indian Healing Tradition by Gopi Warrier and Deepika Gunawant. Element Books (2000).

Ayurvedic Cooking for Self-Healing, 2nd edition by Usha Lad and Vasant Lad. Ayurvedic Press (2006).

Boundless Energy: The Complete Mind–Body Programme for Overcoming Chronic Fatigue by Deepak Chopra. Rider & Co (2001).

B is for Balance

Cancer just loves a body that is out of balance – it gives it so much more opportunity to take control and rampage around. In my experience, the key to fighting back is to keep the body in balance. It is not that easy, but here are a few pointers!

Many complementary therapies that talk about balance are really referring to a balance of energies, or of chakras (see 'A is for Acupuncture'; 'A is for Aromatherapy'; 'A is for Ayurvedic'). This is an extremely common theme. But there are other concepts of balance. We may want to look at how balanced, or imbalanced, our lives are. One way of assessing this is to draw a circle and divide it into sections, each representing a facet of life. How balanced does it look?

Do you take enough (or any) exercise? (The jury is out as to whether hoovering or mowing the lawn counts!) Do you allocate time for your favourite pastime, or perhaps for meditation? Do you take care about what you eat – or is it pit-stop refuelling three times a day, or twice with a substantial input of coffee? Do you have enough rest or 'downtime'?

Dividing the circle and giving yourself points out of ten in each of the important areas of your life can be a good indicator as to if and where there is a problem. It will give you more than a clue as to what professional help you might need to return to a state of balance, to maximize or maintain a state of optimum health, or to put you in the best position to cope with difficult treatments. Whether it be the need for nutritional support, psychological support, a physical trainer, meditation or a complete change of lifestyle – identify the problem and seek some help.

My divided circle was pathetic prior to cancer. But becoming aware of the technique enabled me to see at a glance when the division of my time was not balanced and when my driven personality was on a frolic of its own, wearing out my physical strength and tiring out my spirit. Meditation or 'still time' enabled me to readjust – allowing an inner peace for thoughts to float through (see 'M is for Meditation').

There is also the major issue of nutritional balance, discussed elsewhere in this book, and in great depth by authors such as Patrick Holford.

TOP TIP

Take heed and make time – because your family need *you* to be fit and healthy so you can look after *them*!

Further information
Reference

Say No to Cancer: The Drug-Free Guide to Preventing and Helping Fight Cancer by Patrick Holford and Liz Efiong. Piatkus Books (2010).

B is for Beauty

Beauty, as we all know, is in the eye of the beholder. The question for the person with cancer is how you want to be 'beheld' by others. As my mother used to say, 'You do not necessarily have to *look* how you *feel*.'

There are going to be days when you very definitely are *not* going to feel your best, when even your inner beauty is having a struggle to shine through. So it is essential to look after yourself. Book that haircut, if your treatment allows you to still have hair! Make sure the colour is good – a sharp haircut sets off clothes well and makes it easier to keep looking smart. If you are going to lose your hair (see 'W is for Wigs'), this may be an opportunity to see if blondes really do have more fun!

As far as male readers are concerned, Telly Savalas, star of the 1970s cop series *Kojak* ('Who loves ya, baby?'), completely changed how women view bald men. I have to warn you that there is a whole load of women out there for whom baldness is the ultimate in sexiness. But it has to be a well-cared-for bald head – so lots of rubbing in of almond oil to fend off any dry skin (see 'H is for Hair Loss'). Camomile cream is great for healing rashes. A slight tan is good, and achievable even in the middle of winter with a very gentle fake-tan lotion such as Nivea Body Sunkissed Skin (a hint of self-tan with grapeseed oil) or the Johnson's equivalent from their Holiday Skin range. These do contain some chemicals, so be careful. Apply sparingly, and don't forget to wash your hands immediately to avoid the giveaway brown stains!

Women have many more tools in the make-up box and, after years of disguising hangovers, premenstrual tension (PMT) and other such telling trials, are probably all past mistresses in the Art of Looking Good. Most large department stores offer a free make-up session if you buy a product, just to hone to perfection your artistic talents. Beware of chemicals on the skin (this is another opportunity for reading labels). Fortunately there are now organic product ranges available (see 'Further information'). I can recommend Aveda products which, whilst expensive, seem to last well, and also Yves Rocher and Liz Earle Naturally Active Skincare.

People always say, 'You look so well…' This might be because their expectations are that you are NOT going to look well. I usually answer, 'It just takes SO much longer in front of the mirror!' And everyone laughs. But it is the absolute truth. Sometimes, to look beautiful (or in my case passable) takes an age – so set aside the time for yourself! I make a point of looking particularly 'well' when I visit my doctors. This reinforces my subliminal message about staying as well as possible, tolerating drug regimes and getting on with my extremely enjoyable life even whilst having cancer.

A particular challenge occurred when I was in a drug trial. I was unsure whether it was tackling my liver metastasis, and my skin took on a yellowish hue – often associated with liver cancer. Past panicking about these things, I donned my roll-neck jumper with long sleeves (as it was middle of winter), put gloves on, and added more blusher to my cream foundation. When I saw the research nurse, she said how well I looked. This was followed by the usual questions about the side effects of the drug. I admitted I had no side effects. 'Have you noticed a yellow colour in your urine, which often affects the colour of your skin?' she asked. 'Oh. Obviously not in your case!'

Beauty, of course, is not just about make-up, which will fool only some people, some of the time. It should be a ritual together with good diet, nutrition, exercise and lots of rest – which is difficult to achieve even at the best of times.

Beauty is an integral part of nature. It is uplifting to see and take the time to appreciate the beauty of a natural thing – a rose in bloom with the morning dew, the colours of an autumn leaf, the first snowdrops, the footprints of a fox on a heavy frost. Even on a gloomy day, to find something beautiful is to find inspiration. Seek and you will find.

TOP TIP

Looking good *is* feeling better.

Further information

UK

Aubrey Organics Tel: 0800 0851 697. Website: www.aubreyorganicsuk. co.uk

Liz Earle Naturally Active Skincare Tel: 01983 813913. Website: www. uk.lizearle.com

Aveda Tel: 0800 054 2979. Website: www.aveda.co.uk

Yves Rocher Tel: 0870 049 2222. Website: www.yves-rocher.co.uk

Elena's Nature Collection Ltd Tel: 01435 882092/884090. Website: www.elenasnaturecollection.co.uk

US

Look Good... Feel Better is a free, non-medical, brand-neutral, national public service programme created to help individuals with cancer look good, improve their self-esteem and manage their treatment and recovery with greater confidence. Website: www.lookgoodfeelbetter.org

References

Aveda Rituals: A Daily Guide to Natural Health and Beauty by Horst Rechelbacher. Henry Holt & Company (1999).

Nine Ways to Body Wisdom: Blending Natural Therapies to Nourish the Body, Emotions and Soul by Jennifer Harper. Thorsons (2000).

B is for Biofeedback

There are flows of electricity within the body. One example is the pulses of electricity (derived from the electrical impulses that control the beating heart) which flow through the circulatory system. Research has also established the existence of magnetic fields – again, particularly from the heart, but also from the brain and other muscles in the body. These provide a stream of vibratory information through a continuously interconnected network.

It is suggested that complete health depends on total interconnection and that physical or emotional traumas can lead to an impairment of this connectivity. This in turn reduces the effectiveness of the body's defence and repair systems, allowing disease to take hold. The theory behind biofeedback therapy is that the application of electric and magnetic fields – particularly pulsating magnetic fields – has the potential to restore balance in the vibratory circuits, 'jump starting' the body's own defence and repair systems and facilitating self-healing.

The patient is attached to a safe and non-invasive device which measures the body's stress response to certain Hertz wave frequencies. The frequencies which the body responds to are then fed back in order to encourage self-healing. This can be aimed at relieving the side effects of stresses on the body such as environmental toxins. These would include cancer-fighting drugs and radiotherapy. Biofeedback should therefore support the treatment being given.

TOP TIP

Biofeedback may enhance your body's ability to cope with unhelpful stressors and so support you during treatment and aid in recovery.

Further information
UK
   Linda Crawford Email: linda@allergyline.com. Website: www.allergyline.com

US

For information and help locating qualified providers in the US visit the **Biofeedback Certification International Alliance**: www.bcia.org

References

Energy Medicine: The Scientific Basis by James L. Oschman. Churchill Livingstone (2000).

'Bioelectromagnetics in the service of medicine' by C.A.L. Bassett. This is a chapter in *Electromagnetic fields: biological Interactions and Mechanisms*, edited by Martin Blank. Advances in Chemistry Series 250. American Chemical Society (1995), pages 261–275. A second relevant chapter is 'Therapeutic aspects of electromagnetic fields for soft-tissue healing' by B.F. Sisken and J.Walker.

B is for Biopsy

In a biopsy, a sample of tissue (from a breast lump, for example) is taken for further analysis. This can establish whether or not the suspicious lump or growth is cancerous. It is not a completely foolproof test. It has been known for the person taking the biopsy to miss the lump and take cells from surrounding healthy tissue. But, with increasingly sophisticated guidance from ultrasound scanners, this is becoming a thing of the past. Nevertheless, the accuracy of a biopsy depends on the expertise of the person performing the procedure (which will influence the exact placing of the needle and the amount and quality of the tissue sampled) and the expertise of the person analysing the tissue.

In the case of a breast lump, there are various types of biopsy (but the principles are the same when doctors are investigating other possible cancers).

In fine needle biopsy or aspiration (known as FNA), a syringe attached to the needle is used to remove cells from the lump. These are then smeared onto a slide (as with a Pap smear in screening for cervical cancer) and sent to the lab for analysis. The incidence of false results is 2–5%.

A core (or Tru-Cut biopsy), as the name suggests, takes a larger sample of tissue from the centre of the lump, but this is again done using a needle. It feels like a tiny stun gun. This has now become the gold standard for biopsy, and there are hardly ever false results.

Excision biopsy is sometimes performed when the lump is small, when uncertainty remains about whether or not it is a cancer, and when it can be easily accessed and removed in its entirety. This is usually done without needing a stay in hospital.

In each case, cells, suspect tissue or lumps end up in the path lab, where the tissue is analysed by a specialist pathologist to determine whether or not there is cancer present.

Awaiting the results of a biopsy can be more than a little stressful. It is important to realize that even if the biopsy reveals that cancer is present, there is no need to panic – plenty of time for that later! There are many other tests to be carried out. These include blood tests and perhaps a scan to see if there is any spread to other parts of the body. If that is negative, the next stage will probably be to have the tumour removed surgically.

TOP TIP

Why suffer unnecessarily? Ensure that the person carrying out the biopsy uses a little local anaesthetic. There is usually slight soreness afterwards, and possibly a little bruising. Taking some arnica *before* and after the biopsy may help.

Although the diagnosis in most cases is clear, there are some circumstances – particularly with rare or unusual cancers – when it may be helpful to have a second opinion. If tissue is already available in the lab, there will be no need for another biopsy. Generally, the most accurate results are obtained from centres that see many patients with your particular kind of cancer. In the US, recognition by the National Cancer Institute is a good guide.

Further information
US

An excellent description for patients of the biopsy process can be found at the **CancerGuide** website: www.cancerguide.org/pathology.html

A
B
C
D
E
F
G
H
I
J
K
L
M
N
O
P
Q
R
S
T
U
V
W
X
Y
Z

B is for Blame

Blame is fuelled by anger and is a waste of energy.

Some people consider that their disease is punishment from God. They revisit past sins (real or imagined) to seek God's justification. But is it not great arrogance to speculate as to God's divine purpose? Others seek explanation in the way we have tampered with the world. Or in the way we as individuals have behaved.

A favourite idea is that the harbouring of grudges or resentment can cause disease. And who has not suffered a situation (such as divorce or betrayal) which has caused physical pain or mental angst, and where hurt and bitterness have abounded? It is incredibly depressing when people behave badly or let us down, but there is absolutely no proof that our very human reactions cause cancer, and it is self-defeating to suggest they do. It is good, though, to have a strategy to deal with 'villains'. Do not brood, or play the 'what if' game. Wrap that situation or person in a love bubble and launch the bubble into space where God and the universe will take care of it – while we concentrate our efforts on the positive business of living our lives.

TOP TIPS

Do not be a victim of someone else's villainy.

A little prayer: please help us change the things we can change, ignore the things we cannot change, and grant us the wisdom to know the difference.

Further information
References

Cancer patients are sometimes told that they must maintain a 'positive attitude' to keep their cancer at bay. They may blame themselves if they are unable to do this and their cancer returns. Jimmie Holland, a psycho-oncologist wrote an excellent essay called 'The Tyranny of Positive Thinking' that challenges these assumptions. See www.humansideofcancer.com/chapter2/chapter.2.htm.

The Biology of Belief: Unleashing the Power of Consciousness, Matter and Miracles by Bruce H. Lypton. Hay House UK (2008).

B is for Blessings

There is no better time to count them than when you are diagnosed with or living with cancer.

For my own part, I might never have changed direction – which I recognized I really needed to do – without a diagnosis of cancer. This illness has given me a huge opportunity for personal growth. It has altered my perspective in so many ways.

I am blessed with the most wonderful husband without whose support and strength I probably would have given up. He also has the patience of a saint. Most people who know me think (and some say) that he has to have that to be married to me!

I have changed, and, as I have changed, so too have the people around me – in their views, thoughts and actions.

I have a new day job which really 'floats my boat', and it is writing this book to help others.

Recently, and this has not always been the case, I have really been enjoying my role as sister, auntie and in the wider family. I have always loved being a godmother, but even more so now.

I really know who my friends are, and I have an insight, acceptance and love of humanity, which I had never thought about before. It is a very good feeling of love and being loved.

I have not yet experienced pain. It might come. But at the moment I can count that as a blessing. And I rest content that because of advances in medical care, pain today is not the issue it once was for people with cancer.

I have the blessed and perfect excuse of NOT doing the things I do not want to do.

But, most importantly of all, I have found and talk to my God and Maker – 'Him upstairs' as Auntie Jo used to call Him. I always wondered how such a dynamic and energetic person as Auntie Jo had within her such huge peace, and now I know.

I have been blessed with some time to complete that which I want to complete.

A
B
C
D
E
F
G
H
I
J
K
L
M
N
O
P
Q
R
S
T
U
V
W
X
Y
Z

TOP TIP

Look for the blessing in disguise!

Further information

Reference

Life Is a Gift: The Secrets to Making Your Dreams Come True by Gill Edwards. Piatkus Books (2007).

B is for Bowel (Colorectal) Cancer

The large bowel (made up of the colon and rectum – hence the medical term 'colorectal') is the five-foot long section of intestine through which food remains pass before being expelled through the anus. Certain parts of the digestive tract are especially prone to cancer, and the large bowel is among them: colorectal cancer is the third most common cancer in the UK, and the fourth most common in the United States. The disease is diagnosed in almost 40,000 people each year in the UK, and in 140,000 people in the US. Its incidence differs markedly between different parts of the world and is most frequent where there is a Westernized diet consisting largely of processed foods.

Although the evidence is not entirely consistent, there are reasonable grounds for suggesting that diets rich in fruit, vegetables and cereals reduce the chances of bowel cancer. We are not yet sure why. It could be that people who eat such diets tend to eat less red meat and animal fat (which increase bowel cancer risk). It may have to do with the fact that fruit, vegetables and cereals contain a lot of fibre, which reduces constipation and speeds passage through the bowel of potentially cancer-causing chemicals. Or it could be that such diets are high in protective minerals and vitamins. A further complication is that the benefits of a diet high in fruit and vegetables may be mixed up with the benefits of greater exercise and less obesity (since these factors tend to be found together in people with a healthy lifestyle).

There is little difference in bowel cancer incidence between men and women. Some families have a susceptibility to colorectal cancer, but genetic make-up contributes directly to only a small proportion (perhaps 5%) of the total number of cases. Bowel cancer can develop from a non-cancerous growth called a polyp, so the presence of intestinal polyps is a risk factor. People known to be at particularly high risk can be screened regularly by colonoscopy – an internal examination in which a tiny camera at the end of a flexible fibre optic tube is passed through the anus. (Patients are sedated for this procedure!) There is some evidence that aspirin and related anti-inflammatory drugs reduce the risk of polyps and of colorectal cancer.

A bowel tumour may draw attention to itself through pain and discomfort in the lower abdomen. There could be some alteration in bowel habit, particularly a tendency towards constipation. Discharge of mucus and any bleeding from the rectum are important warning signs. But unless the cancer is towards the very end of the digestive tract, bleeding will not be obvious. Even so, it can be detected by testing stools for 'occult' (i.e. hidden) blood. Screening for bowel cancer using the faecal occult blood test is now being introduced across the UK.

Bowel cancer usually starts as an ulcer in the tissue forming the innermost layer of the intestine. If undetected, it can eventually grow through the full thickness of the bowel wall. It may then spread to nearby lymph nodes and other organs in the pelvis.

Surgery is the main initial treatment for bowel cancer and cures many people who have the disease in its early stages. The operation may involve taking away portions of bowel close to the tumour and local lymph nodes. Colorectal cancer is sensitive to chemotherapy, and drugs can be given after surgery (see 'A is for Adjuvant Therapy') if there is appreciable risk the cancer will return. Radiotherapy can be helpful in shrinking the tumour before an operation or in controlling any cancer that cannot be removed surgically.

A
B
C
D
E
F
G
H
I
J
K
L
M
N
O
P
Q
R
S
T
U
V
W
X
Y
Z

A typical chemotherapy treatment for colorectal cancer that has spread would be fluorouracil given together with leucovorin and either oxaliplatin or irinotecan. The targeted antibody drug Avastin (bevacizumab) is also effective against bowel cancer and can be added to this regimen. (It is approved for treating advanced colorectal cancer in the US but is not available for this purpose on the National Health Service in the UK.) Recently, another antibody drug called cetuximab (Erbitux) has also been shown to slow the progression of bowel cancer when given in combination with chemotherapy.

In later stages of the disease, it is common to find that colorectal cancer has spread through the blood to the liver. It may be possible to remove these liver tumours by surgery. If the secondary cancers are large, chemotherapy can sometimes shrink them sufficiently to allow an operation to go ahead.

Further information

UK

Cancer Research UK: www.cancerhelp.org.uk/type/bowel-cancer

Macmillan Cancer Support: www.macmillan.org.uk/Cancerinformation/cancertypes/Colonandrectum/Colonandrectalcancer.aspx

US

National Cancer Institute: www.cancer.gov/cancertopics/pdq/treatment/colon

Patient Resource Cancer Guide's website has excellent links and resources for people with colon and rectal cancers: http://patientresource.net/colon_and_rectal.aspx

There is also Colon Cancer Alliance: www.ccalliance.org

B is for Brachytherapy

Brachytherapy is used to treat early-stage prostate cancer – that is, when the cancer is confined and has not spread. Radioactive seeds (small radioactive rods about the size of a grain of rice) are implanted via a thin needle into the site of the tumour where they continue to emit radiation for up to a year. Brachytherapy in prostate cancer has several advantages: treatment can be carried out as a day case, the likelihood of it causing urinary incontinence is low, and impotence is less of a risk than with surgical approaches such as radical prostatectomy (see 'P is for Prostate Cancer'). Long-term risks are few, and results show evidence of prolonged disease-free survival. Unlike standard 'external beam' radiotherapy, which can only be delivered once as a course of treatment, brachytherapy may be repeated at the same site. But, as with so many therapies, side effects (such as discomfort passing urine) can be experienced and vary in duration. You may consider integrating some complementary medicine to ease the way.

Whilst brachytherapy is used mostly in prostate cancer, the technique of placing a radiation source next to a target tumour – so delivering a high dose where it is needed while minimizing the exposure of surrounding healthy tissue – is applicable to the treatment of other cancers which are self-contained. In intracavity radiotherapy, a small piece of radioactive material (usually caesium-137) is put next to the tumour. This technique can be used for cancers of the mouth, womb, cervix or vagina.

Further information
UK

The Prostate Cancer Charity, First Floor, Cambridge House, 100 Cambridge Grove, Hammersmith, London W6 0LE. Helpline: 0800 074 8383. General enquiries: 020 8222 7622. Email: info@prostate-cancer.org. uk. Website: www.prostate-cancer.org.uk

Cancer Research UK: www.cancerhelp.org.uk. Follow links from 'Types of treatment' to 'Types of internal radiotherapy'.

US

American Brachytherapy Society: www.americanbrachytherapy.org

B is for Brainwave Therapy (Incorporating EEG Neurofeedback)

This simple therapy uses sound rewards to encourage the brain to produce a healthily balanced ratio of brainwaves. The idea is to create a harmony and balance of emotions that allows the brain to start healing both emotional and physical conditions. The electroencephalogram (EEG) is a recording of the electrical activity of the brain. It is obtained from electrodes placed on the scalp, using a cap and some easily removable glue. When someone is drowsy, electrical activity occurs in regular bursts as groups of cells discharge together. So the EEG waveform is one of large peaks and troughs – a pattern called alpha rhythm. As someone becomes more alert, this pattern is replaced by smaller waves of faster frequency.

By training the individual with EEG neurofeedback, it is possible to reduce stress and depression and thereby to increase health. The key for a cancer patient is to increase the amount of alpha rhythm, since this is a healing state also linked to joy. Although a sort of work-out for the brain, little or no effort is involved.

The technique is completely non-intrusive, relaxing and enjoyable. It is an extremely good tool for dealing with any depression or negativity surrounding a diagnosis of cancer. After an hour's session, I have always felt energized and positive, as well as experiencing a sense of deep inner calm and peace.

Training can work with or without medication. As the brain stabilizes, other modalities can become more effective – and these can range from psychotherapy to drugs. For patients resistant to using medication, brainwave therapy is one of the few options that can help deal with serious problems. No lasting side effects have become apparent during 30 years of research and clinical use.

A survey of psychologists and therapists who use this therapy report three common findings: neurofeedback is commonly used for mood disorders (depression and anxiety) and for attention deficit disorder (ADD)/attention deficit hyperactivity disorder (ADHD); outcomes improve when it is combined with other therapies; and the need for drugs is often reduced.

Over a hundred studies on EEG neurofeedback have been published, and the research is sufficient to encourage a growing number of clinicians and medical schools to adopt the technique.

Further information
UK
Linda Crawford, Bioenergetics and Neurofeedback Practitioner, Hale Clinic, 7 Park Crescent, London W1B 1PF. Tel 020 7631 0156. Email: linda@allergyline.com. Website: www.allergyline.com

US
For information and help locating qualified providers, see the **Biofeedback Certification International Alliance**: www.bcia.org

References
Clinical Efficacy and Cost-Effectiveness of Biofeedback Therapy by R. Schellenberg and colleagues. Association for Applied Psychophysiology and Biofeedback (1989).

Biofeedback by Mark Schwartz and Frank Andrasck. Guilford Press (2005).

The Feeling of What Happens: Body and Emotions in the Making of Consciousness by Antonio Damasio. Harcourt Brace & Co (1999).

'Anxiety change through electroencephalographic alpha feedback seen only in high anxiety subjects' by J.V. Hardt and J. Kamiya. *Science* 1978, volume 201, pages 79–81.

A Guide to Use in Clinical Practice and Research, Minneapolis by W.G. Dahlstrom and G.S. Welsh. An MMPI Handbook, MN University of Minnesota Press (1960).

B is for BRCAI and BRCA2

An inherited form of breast cancer accounts for around 5% of the 45,000 new cases diagnosed each year in Britain. In most of these cases, the defect is in a gene (called BRCA1 or BRCA2) which means that cells do not repair DNA as effectively as normal. In families which carry this genetic mutation, there will usually be a history of women dying early from cancer of the breast or ovary.

Women from such families can now be screened to confirm whether or not they carry the BRCA1 or BRCA2 genes (and two other gene mutations linked to high risk). Among women whose genes do have a mutation, there is an 85% chance of developing breast cancer by the age of 70. One way of dealing with this risk is frequent screening so that any tumour can be removed at the earliest possible stage. Even so, some women choose to have a double mastectomy to prevent the disease developing.

Having a living relative with breast cancer may help in identifying any faulty gene. Before any genetic testing, it is important to have all the relevant information, to consider the impact a positive result might have on you and members of your family, and to think about what you would want to do if a mutation was found.

Further information
UK

Cancer Research UK: www.cancerhelp.org.uk and the Cancer Research UK information nurses. Freephone: 0808 800 4040

Macmillan Cancer Support: www.macmillan.org.uk and their cancer support specialists. Freephone: 0808 808 0000

Breast Cancer Care Freephone: 0808 800 600. This is a government helpline for all enquiries on breast cancer including genetic screening.

US

National Society of Genetic Counselors: www.nsgc.org

FORCE (Facing our Risk of Cancer Empowered): www.facingourrisk.org

Information on Oncotype DX from **Genomic Health**: www.genomichealth.com

Information from **Memorial Sloan-Kettering Cancer Center** on BRCAI and BRCA2: www.mskcc.org/mskcc/html/8623.cfm

B is for Breast Cancer

A
B
C
D
E
F
G
H
I
J
K
L
M
N
O
P
Q
R
S
T
U
V
W
X
Y
Z

More than 45,000 women will be diagnosed with breast cancer this year in the UK. In the US, there will be more than 200,000 new cases. The good news is that the death rate from breast cancer has been falling steadily. In the UK, mortality from breast cancer has declined by 30% over the past two decades and in the US the death rate is dropping by 2% each year. More than 80% of women diagnosed now in the UK can expect to survive at least five years. In the US, the latest estimate is 89% five-year survival. (But it is important to note that breast cancer can recur after five years.)

One reason for this is improved awareness leading to earlier detection of the disease through self-examination and effective screening (see 'M is for Mammogram'). And there have been major advances in treatment due to the development of effective drugs such as tamoxifen and the aromatase inhibitors (see 'A is for Adjuvant Therapy'), trastuzumab (Herceptin) and lapatinib (known as Tykerb in the US and Tyverb in the UK, where the drug is not available on the NHS).

Breast cancer, as with other forms of the disease, is caused by a group of cells behaving badly or, more correctly, abnormally. This clump of cells, which have lost the ability to limit the rate at which they divide, stimulate the body to produce blood vessels and so ensure that they get sufficient oxygen and nutrients to keep on growing.

Finding a lump

All women have been encouraged to self-examine, although there has been considerable debate as to how helpful this really is. It has been suggested, for example, that for women with lumps that disappear and reappear during the monthly cycle, the process can be unnecessarily worrying. It is also far from conclusive. Finding a lump does not necessarily mean cancer:

many are 'benign' (i.e. harmless). And not finding a lump does not necessarily mean there is no breast cancer.

There can be signs other than a lump, such as puckering. But, undoubtedly – for many women – the first worrying indication is detecting a lump that can be anywhere in size from a pea to a duck egg. That is the moment to go for a check-up to the professionals, either your GP or family physician or a One Stop Breast Clinic. If there is any suspicion, the doctor will suggest you have a biopsy: a needle is passed into the lump and some cells are removed for examination under a microscope (see 'B is for Biopsy').

For those whose potential problem is identified because of a screening mammography, this can be the most terrible shock. When you go for your results, be prepared and, ideally, take a friend. In the UK, the Maggie's Centres (see 'M is for Maggie's Centres') offer terrific support if you are lucky enough to have one on the hospital campus. Some hospitals have oncology-trained breast care nurses on hand. The breast clinic should be able to provide information on services available locally, such as counselling.

Being told that it is a cancer

If cancer is confirmed, there is a whole host of questions to ask – and some new terms to learn.

DCIS (ductal carcinoma in situ) means the tumour (carcinoma) has made its home (in situ) in a milk gland (duct). This is generally good news because it means the cancer is happily sitting there and not invading anywhere else. But many cancers are invasive and have spread into breast tissue surrounding the lump or to lymph glands such as those in the armpits.

In my case, the cancer had reached the lymph nodes. One particular lymph node had been very sore indeed. I had thought it was the result of using a new deodorant. But no! The next step is to have more scans (see 'S is for Scans') to see if the cancer has spread elsewhere, such as to the lungs, bones or liver. EVEN IF IT HAS, I can confirm that it is quite possible to be playing tennis and living life to the full with all those cancers and more.

Whatever the outcome of initial treatment, whilst the professionals come up with a personalized master plan for tackling your cancer, YOU must concentrate your efforts on staying and being as well as you can.

Treatment

The size of the tumour will be one factor that determines treatment. So too will be its grade – that is, the degree to which the cells are abnormal. But the most crucial factor is likely to be whether or not there is evidence the tumour has spread within the breast, or to lymph nodes in the armpit, or to nodes and organs elsewhere in the body.

If the tumour is small and still confined to the place where it started to develop, treatment will usually be by lumpectomy rather than removal of the breast (mastectomy). And that might be the last of your brief encounter of the cancer kind. But the surgeon will take tissue from a wide margin around the lump, to see if it contains any cancer cells. And a 'sentinel' lymph node (the one most likely to be reached first by spreading cancer) may be removed for examination in the path lab, to see if it contains any cancer cells.

Surgery will very likely be followed by radiotherapy, designed to reduce the likelihood that the breast cancer will return in the breast or close by. (Effective radiotherapy is the advance that has made breast-conserving surgery possible in so many cases.) Doctors may also advise precautionary treatment with hormone or chemotherapy drugs that circulate around the whole body (see 'A is for Adjuvant Therapy') to prevent tumours developing from any breast cancer cells that have spread to distant sites but are too small to detect by scanning.

Throughout, the key to finding the best treatment is to allow the professionals to identify as much as possible about your cancer. One question will be whether the cells have receptors for the hormone oestrogen. If they do, we know that growth of the cancer is encouraged by oestrogen, and a major aim of any further treatment will be to block the effects of this hormone or cut off its supply. Another question is whether the tumour cells have on them the HER2 growth receptor. If they do, targeted therapy with Herceptin may be helpful. Seeming miracles have been achieved with these new targeted drugs: tumours have shrunk into insignificance in weeks.

Choice of treatment will also be affected by whether you are still clearly premenopausal, going through this period of change or clearly postmenopausal. In premenopausal women, the ovaries are still producing oestrogen. If the cancer is positive for oestrogen receptors, it is important to stop this source of the hormone; this can be done either by surgically removing the ovaries, or through use of drugs called LHRH analogues. Either way, you will experience a sudden menopause and its accompanying symptoms. But using drugs has the advantage that – after two or three years – it is often possible to stop taking them, in which case you may (if still young enough) be fertile once again.

Why do so many women get breast cancer?

Since 1970, breast cancer cases have increased across the age range by around 80%. Among the accepted factors that may account for this increase are trends towards earlier menarche (i.e. the age at which you have your first period), starting a family later in life, less breastfeeding, smaller families, later menopause, HRT, obesity, alcohol consumption and a high-fat diet. A thread linking many of these factors is that they increase the proportion of a woman's life during which oestrogen levels are relatively high.

Among factors that some people think also contribute to the rise in breast cancer are exposure to chemicals in our environment that mimic the effects of oestrogen, fast foods full of preservatives and pesticides, greater exposure to industrial chemicals – a by-product of having more women in the workplace, and the related factor of less time to exercise or relax.

Further information
UK
Cancer Research UK: www.cancerhelp.org.uk/type/breast-cancer/?script=true

Macmillan Cancer Support: www.macmillan.org.uk/Cancerinformation/cancertype/Breast/Breastcancer.aspx

Breakthrough Breast Cancer, Weston House, 246 High Holborn, London WC1V 7EX. Freephone: 08080 100 200. Tel: 020 7025 2400. Website: www.breakthrough.org.uk

US
National Cancer Institute: www.cancer.gov/cancertopics/pdq/treatment/breast

Patient Resource Cancer Guide provides information and a number of useful websites: http://patientresource.net/Breast_Cancer.aspx

References
Dr Susan Love's Breast Book by Susan M. Love and K. Lindsey. Da Capo Press (2010).

What Your Doctor May Not Tell You About Breast Cancer: How Hormone Balance Can Help Save Your Life by John R. Lee, David Zava and Virginia Hopkins. Grand Central Publishing (2005).

Take Charge of your Breast Cancer: A Guide To Getting The Best Possible Treatment by John Link. Owl Books (2002).

Breast Cancer Beyond Convention: The World's Foremost Authorities on Complementary and Alternative Medicine Offer Advice on Healing edited by Mary Tagliaferri, Isaac Cohen and Debu Tripathy. Atria Books (2002).

Your Life in Your Hands: Understanding, Preventing and Overcoming Breast Cancer by Jane Plant. Virgin Books (2006).

B is for Breath and Breathing

We all take breathing completely for granted and think nothing of it. But try the active cycle of breathing technique (ACBT).

Take a deep breath (try to breathe in to the bottom of your stomach). Hold for three seconds then breathe out. Take four regular breaths – then attempt two 'huffs' (that is the blowing out asthmatics will know about since it is used with a peak flow meter). Take regular breaths. Cough. Repeat the exercise every hour.

We know that a panic attack is accompanied by breathlessness. Think about something stressful and you will see how your breathing changes to short staccato breaths as adrenaline kicks in. Conversely, think of yourself in calm and lovely surroundings and you will be aware of the gentle rhythm and steadiness of breathing in and out as the mind, body and spirit find peace.

As it says in chapter two, verse two of Hatha Yoga Pradipika, 'By becoming aware of the nature of the breath and by modifying it, the whole system becomes controlled.'

Fidelma Spilsbury, a Reiki master and yoga teacher, changed my perception of breathing completely. At the time, I had two tumours in the lung and was about to undergo an exploratory lung operation. I also had asthma and a cold and my breathing was irregular and very definitely not calm.

Her teaching and guidance has stayed with me. With her permission, I pass on one of the simplest breathing techniques she uses for beginners.

This is a three-part breath and focuses on the respiratory movements in three parts of the lungs – the clavicle, the thoracic and the diaphragmatic. Concentrate on breathing into those areas individually, while at the same time acknowledging how the respiration is in each region. This will encourage a sense of these body parts. It will also give you a sense of the breathing movements being contracted or expanded in these areas. You can work with these areas separately for several weeks to improve breathing capacity and relax at very deep levels. Special hand positions (called mudras) can be applied to augment the efficacy of breathing movements in each area.

The complete yoga breath is 'breathing into the three areas in one smooth continuous flow'. This is done slowly and steadily by three-quarters filling the lungs, then pausing for a few seconds, before allowing the breath to slowly release. You can either sit in a meditation posture or lie down, whichever is more comfortable, and relax the whole body.

Ujjayi, meaning 'victorious breath' (and sometimes referred to as the psychic breath), is used to calm the mind and deepen the breath. It is usually learnt in three stages but the third stage (although included here) should *not* be attempted when you have any illness or are pregnant as it can overheat the body. None of the stages should be attempted by anyone with severe pulmonary or cardiovascular disorders or high or low blood pressure.

Stage one is creating the 'sound', like the gentle ebb and flow of the sea. Breathe slowly through the nose and allow the breath to move naturally from navel to chest. Relax the tongue and allow it to slide back towards the glottis. This partially closes the glottis and causes the characteristic throat sound, which is also likened to a baby snoring. (To test for the correct sound cover your ears with your hands and breathe normally – that is the same sound.)

Stage two is establishing Puraka (inhalation) and Rechaka (exhalation). Inhale for the count of three; exhale for the count of six so that the exhalation is double the length of the inhalation. Build up to inhaling to the count of four, and exhaling to the count of eight. Do not force the pace: operate within your comfort zone and follow your own rhythm of counting.

Stage three – *which should never be undertaken if you are suffering from any illness or if you are pregnant* – is adding Kumbhaka (retention). Breathe in to the count of four, hold for the count of four and breathe out to a count of eight. Again, build up to this within what is comfortable. Then extend the hold periods: retain for 16, breathing out for eight, and pausing for four.

Each stage should be practised until it is effortless and a feeling of well-being is experienced (see also 'Y is for Yoga').

TOP TIP

One of the quickest ways of sending myself to sleep is to listen to my breathing. I am usually seeking a meditative state in which healing can take place (see 'M is for Meditation').

Further information

UK

Fidelma Spilsbury (Swami Adhyatmananda) of the British Wheel of Yoga taught Anni the breathing techniques outlined above. Fidelma can be contacted on email: fidelma.spilsbury@virgin.net

To find a teacher near you, contact the **British Wheel of Yoga**, the governing body for yoga in the UK. BWY Central Office: British Wheel of Yoga, 25 Jermyn Street, Sleaford, Lincolnshire NG34 7RU. Tel: 01529 306851. Website: www.bwy.org.uk

US

Helpguide: http://helpguide.org/mental/stress_relief_meditation_yoga_relaxation.htm

Stress Relief Exercises site describes deep breathing exercises: www.stress-relief-exercises.com/deep-breathing-exercises.html

References

Asana Pranayama Mudra Bandha by Swami Satyananda Saraswati. Yoga Publications Trust, Munger, India (2008).

The Heart of Yoga: Developing a Personal Practice by T.K.V. Desikachar. Inner Traditions International (1999).

B is for Bristol Approach

See 'P is for Penny Brohn Cancer Care'

C is for Carctol

Carctol is made from eight herbs from the Assam forests in northern India and given as a dietary supplement. Some people claim it can be helpful to cancer patients, but – by the standards used to assess conventional medicines – there is no evidence of benefit. It was discovered by a young Ayurvedic doctor, Nandlal Tiwari, who has been using it for some 20 years. None of the eight ingredients has anti-cancer properties on its own, but the idea is that their *combination* or correct mixture contributes efficacy. In the UK, Carctol can be prescribed by doctors who believe a patient may benefit, but it is not a licensed medicine.

Carctol has received much publicity. But it is difficult to know whether any success attributed to it is due to the herbal mixture itself or to the changes in diet recommended along with it. A non-acidic diet is advised, it is used in conjunction with a digestive enzyme, and you are supposed to drink five litres of water a day. This strategy may contribute to any claimed success. It has been suggested that cancer prefers an acidic state and cannot survive in an alkaline environment (though there is no evidence this is the case). Water flushes out the system and may keep toxins on the move, so the Carctol diet might function as a detox remedy, although again there is at the moment no evidence to support this claim.

Further information

UK

Carctol: www.carctolhome.com

Cancer Research UK: www.cancerhelp.org.uk/about-cancer/treatment/complementary-alternative/therapies/carctol

US

CAM-Cancer's information on Carctol: www.cam-cancer.org/CAM-Summaries/Biologically-Based-Practices/Carctol

C is for Catechins

A
B
C
D
E
F
G
H
I
J
K
L
M
N
O
P
Q
R
S
T
U
V
W
X
Y
Z

Legend has it that the Emperor Shen Nung discovered tea over 5,000 years ago when some tea leaves accidentally drifted into a pot of boiling water, changing its colour. The Emperor appreciated its refreshing and restorative qualities and tea soon became established as a tonic. Later, the taking of tea was elevated to an art form, resulting in the creation of the Japanese tea ceremony, *Cha-No-Yu*, and teahouses. In traditional Chinese and Indian medicine, practitioners use green tea as a stimulant, diuretic and astringent to control bleeding and assist healing. Today, 'a nice cup of tea' is widely known in the UK at least as the panacea for all ills. Growing evidence would suggest there is actually some truth in this claim!

Black, green and oolong teas are derived from the same plant, *Camellia sinensis*. Grown in similar tropical and subtropical climates, the difference between the teas lies in the processing. To produce black tea, the leaves are allowed to oxidize in the sun, which destroys the biologically active polyphenols. In contrast, green tea is produced by lightly steaming the fresh young leaves, preventing oxidation from taking place and thereby preserving these powerfully antioxidant compounds largely responsible for green tea's health benefits. Oolong tea, with a taste more akin to green than black tea, is popular for its reported weight-loss properties and is only partially fermented. Whereas the caffeine content of coffee and black tea is found to inhibit the absorption of vital nutrients and suppress the immune system, green tea, which is lower in caffeine, stimulates immune function.

The specific polyphenols found in green tea are catechins – flavonoid phytochemical compounds that are also found to a lesser extent in black tea, grapes, wine and chocolate. Due to their potent antioxidant, immune-boosting and free radical-neutralizing capabilities, catechins are being investigated for their ability to prevent cancer and heart disease. The primary catechin in green tea (epigallocatechin-3-gallate, or EGCG) is of particular interest: it may be able to suppress tumours by preventing the formation of new blood vessels whilst also blocking an enzyme needed for cancer cells to grow. The Saitama Cancer Research Institute in Japan has reported that women with a history of breast cancer who drank five cups of tea daily were 50% less likely to have a recurrence than women who drank less than five cups. Other research has shown EGCG to be considerably more potent than vitamin C and vitamin E in antioxidant power.

The most promising studies indicating that green tea could reduce the risk of cancers of the breast, prostate, mouth, stomach and bowel have been conducted in Asian countries where green tea consumption is much higher than in the West. It has been suggested that green tea consumption in Japan (which averages three cups a day) is partly responsible for the low levels of cancer found in that country. In 2004, researchers from Perth University published a study showing that men in south-east China who developed prostate cancer were significantly less likely to be green tea drinkers than comparable men who did not develop cancer. The more green tea drunk, the greater the apparent protective effect. This kind of suggestive evidence has led to clinical trials of green tea as a treatment in prostate cancer.

For tea lovers, green tea can be purchased from most health stores and supermarkets in the form of either loose tea or tea bags. By sampling different types of tea such as the evocatively named organic Dragon Well, Gunpowder, Jade Sword and Sencha, you will soon discover your preferred flavour and aroma (see 'Further information'). As boiling water can ruin the taste of a delicate green tea, heating water to 60–70°C is recommended. For those who might find green tea bitter, catechins have been isolated from it and made available in a convenient daily supplement. A dose of around 350 mg would be equivalent to about four cups of green tea.

Note that green tea contains vitamin K, so check with your doctor if you are taking prescription anticoagulants. Green tea may also decrease the effect of the anti-cancer drug bortezomib (Velcade).

TOP TIP

The positive effects of green tea are not limited to internal organs. Used topically as a lotion, it evens out skin tone and wrinkles and protects the skin from damage by ultraviolet light. For detoxing and slimming, try to drink between three and five cups a day.

Further information
UK

JING Tea Ltd, Canterbury Court, London SW9 6DE. Tel 020 7183 2113. Website: http://jingtea.com. Many of this company's tea suppliers have Fairtrade certification. The majority of their teas are Soil Association organically certified.

Healthspan Ltd, PO Box 64, St Peter Port, Guernsey GY1 3BT. Freephone: 0800 73 123 77. Open from 9 a.m. to 6 p.m., seven days a week. Website: www.healthspan.co.uk

Holland and Barrett: www.hollandandbarrett.com

US

Memorial Sloan-Kettering Cancer Center information on green tea: www.mskcc.org/mskcc/html/69247.cfm

Lewis Gale Hospital website's consumer information on green tea. Scroll down to 'Natural and Alternative Treatments' on the main menu and click on 'Herbs and Supplements'. Then find 'Green tea' in the A–Z list: www.alleghany regional.com/healthcontent.asp?page=contentselection/condensed mainindex

Reference

Health Effects of Tea and Its Catechins: Mystery of Tea Catechins by Yukiaki Kuroda and Yukihiko Hara. Springer (2004).

C is for Cat's Claw

Cat's claw (*Uncaria tomentosa*), also known as life-giving vine of Peru, *uña de gato* or hawk's claw, is a woody vine found in the Amazon rainforest. Traditionally, its bark, leaves and roots have been used by the natives of Peru as an anti-inflammatory, anti-tumour and antiviral medicine.

It attracted the attention of the pharmaceutical companies worldwide and their research showed that *Uncaria tomentosa* might help with a list of ailments ranging from cancer to the common cold. In cardiovascular disease, the presence of the anticoagulant rhynchophylline inhibits abnormal blood clotting, so perhaps helping to prevent strokes and other thrombotic conditions (see Rita Elkins' book on the following page).

Cat's claw is a powerful antioxidant that is said to support the immune system and detoxify the intestinal tract. It has been shown in trials to block several inflammatory pathways and works to harmonize the immune system either by boosting underactivity or by modulating one that is stuck in overdrive. Cat's claw is suggested to help friendly, anti-cancer bacteria thrive in the colon.

Uncaria tomentosa is a source of isopteropodine, an alkaloid with properties that support the immune system, proanthocyanidin (Pycnogenol), a powerful antioxidant which scavenges free radicals, and plant steroids stigmasterol and campsterol, which are anti-tumour agents.

It also contains plant sterols proven to have anti-inflammatory properties. It is claimed that cat's claw can give relief from the side effects of chemotherapy, particularly nausea, and it has been used as an adjunctive treatment for cancer and AIDS in Peru and Europe since the early 1990s. *Uncaria tomentosa* water extracts have been shown to enhance DNA repair after chemical-induced damage. Cat's claw is also thought to have anti-cancer activities. Lab results described on the Memorial Sloan-Kettering Cancer Center website (see 'Further information' on the following page) describe growth-inhibitory effects on a range of cancer cells including leukaemia. But the center also notes that no efficacy studies have been carried out in patients.

Cat's claw is available in powder form, compressed tablets or gelatine capsules at most health food stores or naturopathic pharmacies.

A
B
C
D
E
F
G
H
I
J
K
L
M
N
O
P
Q
R
S
T
U
V
W
X
Y
Z

TOP TIP

Check with your doctor that this is compatible with your orthodox regime. Ingredients in cat's claw are broken down by the same liver enzymes that break down many drugs, so – at least in theory – it could alter their efficacy or side effects.

Further information

UK

Dr Rosy Daniel, Health Creation, Bailbrook House, London Road West, Bath BA1 7JD. Helpline: 0845 009 3366. Website: www.healthcreation.co.uk

Penny Brohn Cancer Care: www.pennybrohncancercare.org

US

National Center for Complementary and Alternative Medicine: http://nccam.nih.gov/health/catclaw

Memorial Sloan-Kettering Cancer Center: www.mskcc.org/mskcc/html/69166.cfm

References

'Uncaria tomentosa: Cat's claw' by Philip N. Steinberg. *Health and Healing* February 1997, volume 16.

Cat's Claw: The Rain Forest Herb that Fights Cancer, Relieves Inflammation and Destroys Free Radicals by Rita Elkins. Woodland Publishing (1995).

C is for Causes of Cancer

Just as there are many kinds of cancer, so there are many causes. Factors involved encompass man-made and natural radiation (including the ultraviolet light from the sun that causes skin cancer), chemical agents (such as carcinogens in tobacco smoke), inherited genetic mutations of the kind that may lead to some breast cancers, and certain viruses (such as those that cause cancer of the cervix). None of these agents works in an all-or-nothing fashion, and most increase the risk of only certain types of cancer.

The closest causal link we have between a lifestyle factor and a common cancer is that between smoking and tumours of the lung. About 90% of cases are caused by tobacco. But even a lifelong smoker has less than a 20% chance of developing lung cancer. So there are clearly other factors involved. And smoking has little or no influence on the risk of developing cancers of the colon, breast, skin or brain, for example.

Cancers arise when the DNA of a cell is damaged in a way that destroys its ability to control its own growth. There are many such control mechanisms within a cell, and it almost certainly takes several different episodes of damage to result in cancer. Some of these arise as random genetic mutations when a cell divides. As we become older, the number of times our cells have divided rises, and they are more likely to have accumulated damage. So it is not surprising that the risk of cancer increases steeply with age: almost three-quarters of all cancers occur in people older than 60 years.

Even so, it is thought that about 80% of cancers are caused by environmental factors and are (at least in principle) preventable. This is the word 'environmental' used in a very broad sense that encompasses exposure to carcinogens in the workplace and specific lifestyle habits such as smoking and overindulgence in alcohol (which is now thought to contribute to breast cancer risk, as well as liver cancer). It also includes obesity and diet. The relationship between risk of cancer and what we eat has received much attention. Back in the 1970s, a major study (by Richard Doll and others) compared the frequency of various cancers with dietary habits in 23 countries and concluded that consumption of larger quantities of meat was closely related to increased risk of colon cancer, and fat intake to cancer of the breast.

The contribution made by lifestyle and environmental factors to risk of breast cancer is illustrated by the experience of Japanese women who moved to the United States. The breast cancer incidence in Japan is lower than in America. But in Japanese women living in the US, risk of the disease is roughly the same as that among American women.

You can help avoid cancer by:

- not smoking
- eating plenty of fruit and fresh vegetables

- avoiding fatty meat (eat lean or white meat)
- taking plenty of exercise
- not getting fat
- avoiding excess alcohol (but a glass or two is fine)
- avoiding unprotected casual sex
- not getting sunburned
- accepting screening when invited (for cancer of the cervix, breast and colon).

Further information

UK

Macmillan Cancer Support: www.macmillan.org.uk/Cancerinformation/ Causesriskfactors/Causes

Cancer Research UK: http://info.cancerresearchuk.org/cancerand research/learnaboutcancer

US

National Cancer Institute, Cancer causes and risk factors: www.cancer. gov/cancertopics/causes

Physicians' Committee for Responsible Medicine, Commentary on Cancer Prevention: www.pcrm.org/resources/education/nutrition/nutrition 2.html

The Cancer Project explores factors contributing to the development of cancer, including dietary factors: www.cancerproject.org/diet_cancer/ index.php

C is for Chemicals

See also 'P is for Pesticides'

Even the water we drink from our taps is full of chemicals. Legislation currently permits levels of contaminants which do not ostensibly constitute a threat to public health – but how good can *any* contaminants be? Fluoride, added to support dental health, has been controversial for many years. There have also been worries about chlorine, nitrates and heavy metals. For a cancer patient, these chemicals can contribute to chemical overload. Pure water is my preferred choice. Chemicals from plastic water bottles can apparently leach into the water, especially if left in the sun! So water in glass bottles is the purist's approach.

But the worst ingress of chemicals into our system is through the food that we eat. One way of bringing this to a firm halt is to eat only organic food and cease eating anything processed. I include in that category anything pre-packed, tinned or microwavable. The vast array of chemicals used in beauty products, and the more expensive creams in which in the past I have indulged, are a concern.

Chemicals were not an issue for me until I was diagnosed with cancer. I then realized that if I wanted to prolong my life, there was no escape from chemotherapy. I thought I would tolerate my treatment better if I eliminated all other chemicals. I spent a huge amount of time in supermarkets reading labels and realized we live in a world full of chemicals – in bath cleaners, dishwasher tablets, toothpaste, hair shampoo, colourants, deodorants, etc., etc. The shopping list below gives some eco-friendly alternatives.

If you are a label reader, look out for formaldehyde (which is a metabolite of the sweetener aspartame), ammonia, sodium hydroxide, sodium bisulphate, naphthalene, chlorine and muriatic hydrochloric acid. What's in this Stuff? by Pat Thomas provides much more information on this subject and is a 'must have' book. She has a host of 'try this instead' ideas which offer real alternatives (see 'References' on the following page).

Even the essential oils used in aromatherapy can be chemically concocted. Why would one want to do this when the natural plant-based product is available? Think, and read the label.

There are also chemicals in the air that we breathe as we walk along the pavement by a busy road or past the dry cleaners! It is extraordinary how the sense of smell becomes more acute to chemical products. A trip to the hairdresser for me is an ordeal because of the airborne chemical smells, particularly if the salon carries out manicures at the same time. Sadly no one has yet produced a chemical-free nail polish and in the summer even I succumb.

TOP TIP

Our bodies are so overloaded with chemicals that it is no wonder our immune systems cannot cope.

Read the labels. Follow the NCIML (No Chemicals In My Life) regime.

Further information

UK

For further information on pesticides and chemicals see **Food Standards Agency**: www.eatwell.gov.uk/healthissues/factsbehindissues/pesticides and www.food.gov.uk/safereating/chemsafe/pesticides

For information about food labelling see **Food Standards Agency**: www.food.gov.uk/foodlabelling

Soil Association: www.soilassociation.org

Fortunately, chemical-free nail polishes are now available. **Inspirationail** is a UK-based company specializing in non-toxic nail varnishes that are free of DBP, formaldehyde and toluene: www.inspirationail.com

US

For a list of foods that contain the most pesticides and chemicals see **The Greenest Dollar**: www.thegreenestdollar.com/2009/06/which-foods-have-the-most-chemical-pesticides

Products certified as 95% or more organic bear a label that says USDA Organic. This link from the **Mayo Clinic** describes labelling practices: www.mayoclinic.com/health/organic-food/NU00255

For further information from the **National Agriculture Library** follow the 'Food Labelling' link at: http://riley.nal.usda.gov

References

What's in this Stuff? The Hidden Toxins in Everyday Products and What You Can Do About Them by Patricia Thomas. Perigee Books (2008).

Say No to Cancer: The Drug-Free Guide to Preventing and Helping Fight Cancer by Patrick Holford and Liz Efiong. Piatkus Books (2010). I particularly recommend this book as essential reading. Much of what Patrick says is backed up by serious academic research and the notes make fascinating reading: www.patrickholford.com.

The Safe Shopper's Bible: A Consumer's Guide to Household Products, Cosmetics and Food by David Steinman and Samuel Epstein. John Wiley & Sons (1995). Contains some good tips but mostly lists products available in the American market.

The Toxic Consumer: How to reduce your exposure to everyday toxic chemicals by Karen Ashton and Elizabeth Salter-Green. Impact Publishing (2007).

C is for Chemoembolization

This technique involves delivering chemotherapy drugs to the site of the tumour through blood vessels which are then blocked. This traps the drugs where they are needed to kill cancer cells while preventing them from circulating around the body as a whole. For example, when a liver cancer cannot be removed by surgery, one established technique is to inject chemotherapy into the hepatic artery that serves the liver and then block it with small gelatin capsules. This targeted approach allows high doses to be delivered to the tumour while avoiding many of the side effects that result from having toxic drugs circulating around the whole body. Even so, side effects such as nausea, vomiting, pain and a high temperature (lasting for two or three days) are possible.

If the cancer returns, chemoembolization can be repeated in a way that radiotherapy and systemic chemotherapy often cannot. There are other forms of local therapy for cancer, such as implanting radioactive wire or seeds close to or inside the tumour (see 'B is for Brachytherapy').

Further information
UK
Cancer Research UK information on chemotherapy for liver cancer: www.cancerhelp.org.uk/type/liver-cancer/treatment/chemotherapy-for-liver-cancer

US
Radiological Society of North America and American College of Radiography: www.radiologyinfo.org/en/info.cfm?pg=chemoembol

C is for Chemotherapy

See also 'D is for Drugs'

In many people's minds, the mere word 'chemotherapy' conjures up an idea of the worst possible poisonous treatment. In the 1950s it probably was. But things have moved on,

A
B
C
D
E
F
G
H
I
J
K
L
M
N
O
P
Q
R
S
T
U
V
W
X
Y
Z

and it is important not to be swayed by the myth. Recognize chemotherapy for what it is: in many cases a life-saving treatment. Among the most striking examples of this are testicular cancer, Hodgkin's disease and childhood leukaemia, where cure rates are now 80–90% (and, for testicular cancer, even higher). In these cases, chemotherapy (allied in many cases to surgery and radiotherapy) eliminates the tumour, and it does not return. So, when considering your treatment options, do not rule out chemotherapy.

The hallmark of cancer cells is that they reproduce rapidly. Chemotherapy kills cancer cells by stopping cell division. But, since healthy cells also divide – albeit at a slower rate – they too can be damaged by anti-cancer drugs. The normal cells that are worst affected are those that divide relatively rapidly. Such cells are found in the bone marrow, where they form the components of blood, in the hair follicles and skin, and in the lining of the intestines. Hence the main side effects of chemotherapy are depletion of white blood cells and anaemia, hair loss and skin ulcers, and nausea and vomiting. Fortunately, the past two decades have seen important advances in our ability to prevent and treat most of these adverse effects. Growth factors can be given to stimulate production of blood cells, and there are now drugs (anti-emetics) that very effectively reduce nausea and vomiting.

Chemotherapy drugs are usually given by an injection into a vein (intravenous administration), but some are available in tablet form. There are various techniques for intravenous injection. One is to deliver drugs through a small tube, or cannula, inserted into a vein on the back of the hand. Drugs can also be infused into a vein close to the heart. This is reached through a thin tube (or catheter) inserted under the skin of the chest and into a vein near the collarbone, or through a vein near the elbow. The frequency of treatment varies: some regimes are weekly, others every three weeks or every month. There are more than 50 different chemotherapy drugs, and side effects vary from one to another.

There are many myths and untruths circulating about this form of treatment. I was minded not to have chemotherapy under any circumstances, but it was suggested that I should at least give it a try. For some people, it is a walk in the park, I was told, and if I did not like it, I could stop. This was enough to get me through the door, into the room, sitting down and having my chemotherapy. And, guess what? It was a walk in the park.

My hair fell out with my first round of the frontline chemotherapy concoction of Adriamycin and fluorouracil. I was devastated about the hair loss but I did not feel at all sick. The second round resulted in a sore mouth and tired legs – usually after I had been overdoing it. This was easily brought under control with a few early nights and some home pampering. It's a good idea to stay away from citrus fruit and to drink loads of water. I did have one black nail and can recommend solar oil or neat vitamin E oil rubbed into the nails at night.

Loss of appetite was never an issue for me. If anything, I felt even more deserving of nice non-slimming treats such as a Kit Kat with tea. But if one does experience loss of appetite, this is the perfect opportunity to change dietary habits.

Of the techniques for giving chemotherapy, I very much preferred cannulation. This requires a high level of expertise from the nursing staff who must select a good vein on the back of the hand – then blood can be taken and chemotherapy given all from the same location. The cannula is taken out at the end of the treatment and a sticking plaster for a few hours is all that is required.

Some people are happier having chemotherapy in the company of a friend. I preferred to be on my own. I used the time for myself and took a book I wanted to read but hadn't had time to. I found that soothing music worked and I usually fell asleep until it was all over. I woke completely relaxed and then tried to stay in that state while I headed for home and bed. I tried to do nothing that evening but sleep it off. For those of you with a meal to prepare, this is the moment to call a friend.

A key side effect that needs careful watching is the reduction in the number of white cells in the blood. This lowers resistance to infection. There are herbal remedies such as echinacea and other products claimed to boost the immune system, such as IP6 (see 'I is for IP6 and Inositol'). Whatever you take, *it is very important* to check it out first with your hospital pharmacy and doctor to ensure that it is not in conflict with your drug regime.

Take all other chemicals that you can out of your life. And make sure that when you are having chemotherapy you are totally relaxed. Breathing exercises are good for this (see 'B is for Breath' and 'V is for Visualization'). If you have a television by your chair or bed, do not be tempted to watch any violent films, because you become tense without realizing it. Be as happy as you can under the circumstances.

Many complementary therapies are available to support one through chemotherapy. They can help with relaxation (see 'A is for Aromatherapy' or 'R is for Reflexology (or Reflex Zone Therapy)') or combat side effects (see 'N is for Nausea'). Patrick Holford (see 'References' on the following page) has a chapter entitled 'Maximizing Recovery', which gives a protocol for nutritional support during and after chemotherapy and radiotherapy.

TOP TIP

To keep well through chemotherapy, you have to focus on your own well-being – and so does everyone else! This is a big pamper opportunity!

Further information

UK

Penny Brohn Cancer Care's information about natural approaches to dealing with the side effects of treatment: www.pennybrohncancercare.org

US

Whilst the information at the link below was written for lymphoma patients, the tips on preparing for chemotherapy and getting through treatments apply to most chemotherapies. See **Patients Against Lymphoma**: www.lymphomation.org/chemo-support.htm

References

Say No to Cancer: The Drug-Free Guide to Preventing and Helping Fight Cancer by Patrick Holford and Liz Efiong, Piatkus Books (October 2010).

The Chemotherapy and Radiation Therapy Survival Guide: Information, Suggestions and Support to Help You Get Through Treatment by Judith McKay, Nancee Hirano and Myles E. Lampenfeld. New Harbinger (1998).

C is for Choices

To live or to die.

To live as well as possible for as long as possible.

Refusal to surrender to fear will transcend fear.

Refuse to suffer pain.

My personality and spirit will win through.

To set an example to others – death is a part of life.

Is the knife the answer/only option?

Breast – mastectomy or not, with reconstruction now or reconstruction later?

Is there a new targeted therapy available (such as Herceptin) or am I stuck with traditional chemo?

Is radiation an option? If so, what type?

TOP TIP

The choices are yours.

C is for Clinical Trials

Clinical trials are conducted in all branches of medicine and they have contributed greatly to advances in care. Their purpose is to provide an objective, unbiased assessment of the benefits and risks of new drugs or other interventions. This is achieved by allocating patients at random either to the new treatment or to a control group which receives standard care. Both groups are followed carefully, and information is collected about efficacy and side effects.

Because the expectations of both patients and doctors can affect outcome, clinical trials are designed – whenever possible – so that neither the doctors giving the treatments nor the patients receiving them know which group they are in until a code is broken at the end of the study. This is called a double-blind trial. Where only the patients are unaware of the treatment given, the trial is single-blind. If there is no standard drug treatment against which to compare a new agent, patients in the control arm are given a dummy (or 'placebo') pill which looks like the active one but contains only inert ingredients.

From a patient's perspective, taking part in a clinical trial is an opportunity to have drugs that are not otherwise available. Being on a trial ensures that you will be carefully monitored before, during and after treatment, so you will have rather more extensive tests and more attention given to you and your case. Of course there is a 50–50 chance of having the control treatment rather than the new one. But since the new treatment has not yet been proved superior to the old one (and indeed it may not be any better), that may not matter.

Any trial you might be considering will be very clearly explained to you in person, and there will be written information you can take away and look at, perhaps together with your family. Whatever your decision, there is no stigma attached, or indeed pressure of any kind. It is important to be very sure that you want to take part. You are allowed to withdraw at any time, which is only fair, even though too many withdrawals could jeopardize the accuracy of a trial's results.

The logistics of taking part must be considered prior to volunteering. Will you be able to travel to a hospital which is not readily accessible? Will there be too many constraints on your time? Might you have unexpected side effects to contend with?

TOP TIP

Some trials are complicated and use sophisticated drug combinations; others are extremely simple. There may be one that suits you.

Further information
UK

The **Cancer Research UK** website has a section on clinical trials which can be searched by tumour type: www.cancerhelp.org.uk

The section on cancer treatments on the **Macmillan** website allows you to search for clinical trials. Follow the link from cancer information: www.macmillan.org.uk

US

www.clinicaltrials.gov is a website run by the **United States National Institutes of Health**. It has very good introductory sections explaining the purpose of trials and how they are conducted and also lists thousands of ongoing trials by tumour type. Some are recruiting patients only in America, but many of the most important studies of new treatments take patients from countries all over the world.

Your doctor may not mention all trials available for your type of cancer, so it can be helpful to investigate available options on your own.

Centerwatch is a global source of clinical trial information offering news, analysis, study grants, career opportunities, and trial listings to professionals and patients. You tell them your type of cancer and they inform you of appropriate trials via email: www.centerwatch.com

If you call 1-800-4-Cancer, you can talk with staff, describe your tumour type, stage, etc. They will then send you a pack containing information on trials that you might be eligible for. Sites that provide information on particular kinds of cancer may also help you find trials. The **Lymphoma Research Foundation**, for example, provides this service to patients: www.lymphoma.org

For questions to ask your doctor about clinical trials, see **Time Magazine**: www.time.com/time/covers/1101020422/questions.html

C is for Coenzyme Q10

The body makes its own Coenzyme Q10, but stress or illness can deplete the supply. Its role is to support the healthy function of cells and the immune system. As it is a powerful antioxidant (see 'A is for Antioxidant Vitamins and Minerals'), CoQ10 protects the fats in membranes from being oxidized by free radicals.

A
B
C
D
E
F
G
H
I
J
K
L
M
N
O
P
Q
R
S
T
U
V
W
X
Y
Z

It is suggested that CoQ10 prevents brain cell deterioration, but most of the research focuses on its contribution to the health of the heart. This has clear relevance to breast cancer patients who have been treated with a chemotherapy drug called Adriamycin (doxorubicin) which can be toxic to the heart, particularly if combined with Herceptin (trastuzumab). The National Cancer Institute website concludes that clinical trials have demonstrated a cardioprotective effect from CoQ10 in patients treated with doxorubicin, but another authoritative review came to the conclusion that there is no overall evidence of benefit. Studies investigating the direct beneficial effect of CoQ10 on breast cancer have not conclusively demonstrated a major anti-cancer effect.

There is another situation in which Coenzyme Q10 supplements may have a potentially useful role. Statin drugs, taken to lower blood cholesterol and so risk of heart disease and stroke, reduce levels of CoQ10 because they inhibit its production by the body. It has not yet been proved that people taking statins benefit from extra intake of this enzyme, but that is a distinct possibility.

TOP TIP

As with any endeavour to integrate herbs, vitamins or antioxidants, it is absolutely essential that you discuss the implications of taking CoQ10 with your oncology team. There may be a timing issue – such as not taking it during chemotherapy or radiotherapy – or there may be contraindications given your existing medication. So *check first.*

Further information
UK

For evidence-based information see **National Health Service**: www.library. nhs.uk/cam

Penny Brohn Cancer Care: www.pennybrohncancercare.org

US

In the United States, no government agency is responsible for routinely testing CoQ10 or ubiquinol supplements for their contents or quality. Both can be highly variable. **ConsumerLab** is an organization that tests supplements to determine if they contain what is claimed and evaluates products for contaminants: www.consumerlab.com

References

Nutrition and Cancer: State-of-the-Art by Sandra Goodman. Health Research Ltd (2003). Order from www.drsgoodman.com/books-goodman.

'Support of drug therapy using functional foods and dietary supplements: Focus on statin therapy' by S. Eussen and colleagues. *British Journal of Nutrition* 2010, volume 103, pages 1260–1277.

C is for Cold Cap

Most chemotherapies are targeted at killing fast-growing cells. The problem is that the chemotherapy cannot distinguish between the fast-growing cells of the cancer and those of the hair follicles. In extreme cold, the blood capillaries contract to reduce blood flow and so preserve the body's warmth. The idea of using a cold cap is to try and prevent the blood carrying the chemo from reaching the hair follicles, thereby saving the hair from falling out. That's the theory!

The cold cap is like an insulated, old-fashioned swimming hat which is completely frozen and placed on one's head about half an hour before chemotherapy. A new frozen cap is brought approximately every 40 minutes through the chemotherapy and once after it.

Extremists like me even wore frozen eye pads in an attempt to keep eyebrows and eyelashes. So I looked a bit like old pictures of Amy Johnson – definitely not for my public! The first three minutes are completely excruciating. I have never felt such cold and I really thought I was not going to be able to bear it. My very strict (and good) friend had told me that if others could do it, I could. I was thinking about how I was going to explain to her that I'd given up after the first few seconds when the three minutes were over and the completely unbearable cold had subsided into cold that was just about bearable. It was rather like being on deck on a boat sprayed with icy water – or being stuck on a ski button with a full-on ice blizzard in the face. Since these are situations I find myself in for fun, the chemotherapy department, with its total lack of wind chill, suddenly took on an almost sunny clime.

I did lose my hair, and it was just starting to grow through again when I started a new regime of paclitaxel with Herceptin. The first infusion was to be given over five hours and I was determined to give not losing my hair, eyebrows and eyelashes the best possible chance. So I had cold caps every half hour throughout the session, for six hours in total. And I did not lose my hair! Do not be deterred – you too can do it. Try and transport your mind somewhere else. Divert your attention with a good book, or if, like me, the ability to concentrate is much diminished with extreme cold, try a video or DVD. Or just allow yourself to drift off to sleep. Do not despair if your hair falls out. For men it's very sexy, and for women – see 'W is for Wigs'. There is one definite up-side – the smoothest hair-free legs!

TOP TIP

Take an aspirin and slightly wet your hair so that the cold cap freezes to your head. A warm towel or blanket around the back of your neck at the same time as the cold cap on your head works wonders.

C is for Colonic Irrigation (or Colonic Hydrotherapy)

Colonic hydrotherapy is an 'internal bath'. It cleanses the colon (the last five feet of the digestive tract) and rids it of deposits that could have been there since childhood. Filtered water introduced through the anus aids the softening, release and expulsion of faecal matter and more compacted toxic deposits.

Before I was diagnosed with cancer, I felt perfectly well in my completely toxic state. As I gathered knowledge, I realized that my system was overloaded with chemicals. By taking the chemicals out of my life, by eating no dairy products or red meat, and by drastically cutting my alcohol and chocolate consumption, I knew I was giving myself the best chance of standing up to the treatments I would be having. Even then, it was not until I had taken part in a clinical trial where the drugs had some very unpleasant side effects (including spots in the mouth, eyes and skin) that I felt sufficiently brave (or desperate) to try this form of detoxification.

Further information
UK

Pure Colonics, The Berkeley Centre, 3 Berkeley Square, Clifton, Bristol BS8 1HL, member of International Association of Colonic Hydrotherapists. Tel: 07900 984584. Email: info@purecolonics.co.uk. Website: www.purecolonics.co.uk

Physical and Emotional Detoxification Programme, The Holistic Healing Centre, Lynden Hill Clinic, Linden Hill Lane, Kiln Green, Nr. Twyford, Berkshire RG10 9XP. Tel: 0118 940 1234. Website: www.lynden-hill-clinic.co.uk

Shymala Ayurveda, 152 Holland Park Avenue, London W11 4UH. Tel: 020 7348 0018. Email: enquiries@shymalaayurveda.com. Website: www.shymalaayurveda.com

The Clifton Experience Colonic Hydrotherapy Email: enquiries@thecliftonexperience.co.uk

References

'Colonic hydrotherapy for intestinal cleansing' by Emma Lear, *Positive Health*, May 2006, page 38.

For a sceptical view, see *Your Friday Dose of Woo: Mere regularity is not enough* at http://scienceblogs.com/insolence/2006/07/your_friday_dose_of_woo_mere_regularity_1.php.

C is for Colorectal Cancer

See 'B is for Bowel Cancer'

A
B
C
D
E
F
G
H
I
J
K
L
M
N
O
P
Q
R
S
T
U
V
W
X
Y
Z

C is for Complementary Therapy

See 'A is for Alternative and Complementary Therapy'

C is for Control

Expressions such as 'taking control' or 'having a sense of control' suddenly appear in the language used about a condition like cancer. This reflects the disease itself: the nature of cancer is that cells are out of control. They have been having a gay old time without you being aware of it. Various strategies can be empowering.

When first diagnosed, most people react – like the rabbit in the headlights – with shock and terror. As the notion of having cancer becomes more familiar, there seem to be two kinds of response. One group does not want to be in control, and the other does. There are people who simply do not want to engage with the problem. They would rather have the doctor, oncologist or other specialist take control and tell them what to do. Then, they hope – like a bad dream – it will pass. Others want to know everything about the disease and have a full briefing from the experts before coming to their own decisions about treatment. Both attitudes are completely normal and understandable.

Medical specialists also fall into two groups. There are those who do not want too many time-consuming questions and wish patients would get on with it and do as they are told. Such doctors sometimes resort to trying to scare you with a meaningless statistic or a threatening 'if you don't do this, then such and such will happen...' sort of statement. The second group goes to huge lengths to make sure you fully understand, encourages you to engage with the issues, stands by you and helps in making choices that are right for you. I am convinced both groups really care about their patients. It is just a matter of different styles. Perhaps the most important aspect of a patient having control is that they choose the doctor that is right for them.

The usual reason for patient complaints is not the individual member of staff, but the huge workload imposed by the overburdened National Health Service. Even so, while not being confrontational, you owe it to yourself to be satisfied and happy about your care. You can ask to be seen or treated by someone else. It is your choice, your right and in your control (see also 'E is for Exceptional or Expert Patient').

TOP TIP

Even if you feel your cancer is spiralling out of control and all is lost, you can still exercise choice. Unpack the various aspects of your life. Is your diet mostly fatty and processed foods? Change to organic. Is your lifestyle one of late nights and lots of alcohol? Change to nurturing, early nights with as much pampering as possible. These are examples of taking control.

Further information
UK
Penny Brohn Cancer Care: www.pennybrohncancercare.org

References

Love, Medicine and Miracles by Bernie Siegel. Rider & Co (1999).

Everything You Need to Know to Help You Beat Cancer by Chris Woollams. Health Issues Ltd (2005).

Challenging Cancer: Fighting Back, Taking Control, Finding Options (2nd edition) by Maurice Slevin and Nira Kfir. Class Publishing (2002).

C is for Cryotherapy

Cryotherapy (or cryosurgery) is used as an alternative to conventional surgery, radiation and drugs for certain types of cancer. It has proven success as a treatment for some prostate, renal and liver cancers – both as initial therapy and if the cancer has returned. The technique is also being studied in lung cancer and as a possible alternative to lumpectomy in small early breast cancers. Cryotherapy has shown particular promise in relieving pain when tumours are located in bone.

Cryotherapy or cryosurgery uses ultrasound images to help the doctor guide needle-like probes through the skin until they penetrate the tumour. Then argon gas is pumped through the probes where it is compressed and expanded resulting in a huge temperature drop (minus 180°C can be achieved). This causes an ice ball to form around the tumour. The ice ball is then thawed with the application of helium gas. The freeze and thaw cycles are repeated to gain maximum effect. The dead tumour tissue is absorbed by the immune system.

Recently, there have been some especially encouraging results from a Canadian study which showed that cryosurgery for localized prostate cancer controlled the disease just as well as radiotherapy over a period of four years. A potentially even more exciting development is cryo-immunotherapy. Using the same probe system that destroys the bulk of the tumour by cryoablation, it is possible to introduce an immune therapy (see 'V is for Vaccines') straight to the site of the problem with the aim of helping the body's immune system deal with any remaining cancerous cells.

Cryotherapy is minimally invasive and can generally be carried out as a day surgery procedure, reducing the need for hospitalization and convalescence required by more invasive techniques. At present there are about 40 hospitals in the UK treating cancer with cryotherapy.

TOP TIP

Investigate this – it could be the future.

Further information
UK

The Prostate Cancer Charity: www.prostate-cancer.org.uk/information/treatment/treatment-choices/cryotherapy

Cancer Research UK: www.cancerhelp.org.uk/about-cancer/cancer-questions/cryotherapy-for-prostate-cancer

US

National Cancer Institute, *Cryosurgery in Cancer Treatment: Questions and Answers*: www.cancer.gov/cancertopics/factsheet/Therapy/cryosurgery

American College of Radiology and Radiological Society of North America, cryotherapy explained: www.radiologyinfo.org/en/info.cfm?pg=cryo

Reference

The Male Lumpectomy: Focal Therapy of Prostate Cancer by Gary Onik and Karen Barrie. AuthorHouse (2005).

C is for Crystal Healing

Crystals and stones have been associated with healing since the beginning of time. The earliest records of crystal healing come from ancient Egyptian, traditional Chinese and Indian Ayurvedic medicine. This complementary therapy aims to restore health to mind, body and spirit using crystals to heal through vibration and resonance by realigning the 'chakras' or 'energy centres' and correcting imbalances which can cause disease.

Chakras are thought to control the health of specific areas of our body and are associated with our physical, mental and emotional interactions. A blockage in 'life force', '*qi*' or 'prana' in one of the seven major chakras can affect all the others. Every crystal and gemstone has its own different vibration of mineral energy, believed to correspond to the vibrational energy of each specific chakra. Crystal healing is often associated with powerful changes to our energy vibrations and fundamental way of being, resonating with the chakras to relieve stress and tension and promote relaxation, peace, harmony and revitalization.

Much belief and folklore is based on the physical characteristics of a stone or crystal, with its colour, rather than its vibrational strength and frequency, suggesting its association with a particular chakra. For example, tiger's eye became associated with courageous tiger-like characteristics and clear-sightedness – both literally and figuratively – whilst the iridescent moonstone, which when polished allows light to show as a crescent in the stone, evokes qualities of clarity and intuition.

During a typical session, the therapist will place a few small crystals on or around you and through them channel healing. For example, amethyst is used to help relieve headaches or stress, rose quartz for enhancing your body's ability to heal and black tourmaline for inner strength and assertiveness.

Another suggested crystal healing technique is to make an elixir or essence by first identifying the attributes of the crystal you need, then selecting and immersing the crystal in water for the required time before drinking.

Central to the understanding of crystal therapy is the belief that the free flow of energy through and around layers of the subtle biomagnetic energy field (or aura) surrounding our physical body is essential to our mental, spiritual and physical well-being. Contemplated for thousands of years, only relatively recently has science proven that every living organism is in fact surrounded by an electromagnetic field. Naturally this has greatly enhanced the credibility of crystal healing as an holistic therapy.

TOP TIP

Try it and see!

If you are experiencing any swelling or inflammation you might like to try wearing a bracelet incorporating malachite, an ore of copper. Malachite allows the body to absorb tiny amounts of copper and is known to alleviate these symptoms.

Further information
UK
British Crystal Healers (BCH) is the leading body for crystal healing in the UK for practitioners who have qualified through the Affiliation of Crystal Healer Organizations or Crystal Healing Federation: www. britishcrystalhealers.org

For practitioners in your area see the **Crystal and Healing Federation** website: http://new.crystalandhealing.com, or **The Healing Trust**: www.thehealingtrust.org.uk

References

The Crystal Bible: A Definitive Guide to Crystals by Judy Hall. Godsfield Press (2003).

The Crystal Bible, Volume 2 by Judy Hall. Godsfield Press (2009).

Crystal Power Crystal Healing: The Complete Handbook by Michael Gienger. Cassell Illustrated (2005).

The Essential Crystal Handbook: All the Crystals You Will Ever Need for Health, Healing and Happiness by Simon and Sue Lilly. Duncan Baird (2006).

The Complete Guide to Crystal Chakra Healing: Energy Medicine for Mind, Body and Spirit by Philip Permutt. CICO Books (2009).

The Element of Harmony written and published by Nat and Tony Bondar (2004): www.crystalharmony.co.uk.

C is for Curcumin

Curcumin is found in turmeric, the yellow spice used in curries. It has been part of both Ayurvedic and Chinese medicine for centuries. It is suggested that curcumin has many different ways of interfering with cancer. It is a powerful antioxidant and so reduces the amount of free radicals circulating in the body. Work in the laboratory suggests that curcumin supports the immune system and could protect the body against the effect of toxic chemicals and other agents (including chemotherapy and radiotherapy). It encourages damaged cancer cells to self-destruct (a process called apoptosis) and may make it more difficult for tumours to grow, develop their own blood supply and spread through the body.

Curcumin is in clinical trials in patients with cancer of the pancreas and colon and in several malignant blood disorders. It is also being assessed in autoimmune conditions such as psoriasis and in patients with Alzheimer's disease. There is a proviso that it cannot be mixed with some chemotherapies and high doses of certain food supplements.

TOP TIPS

Boil a large teaspoon of turmeric with a red onion in half a pint of water for a simply delicious drink.

In the US, the organization ConsumerLab has found problems (including contamination) with certain curcumin supplements. They issue lists of products that have passed their tests (www. consumerlab.com/reviews/Turmeric_Curcumin_Supplements/ Turmeric).

Natural curcumin may not be well absorbed by the body and work is underway to develop versions of the substance which could provide a more reliable beneficial effect.

Further information
UK

An article on findings published in the **British Journal of Cancer** indicating the possibility that natural chemicals found in turmeric could be developed into new treatments for oesophageal cancer: 'Curry spice "kills cancer cells"' (October 2009) http://news.bbc.co.uk/1/hi/8328377.stm

Cancer Research UK, 'Can turmeric prevent or treat cancer?': www. cancerhelp.org.uk/about-cancer/cancer-questions/can-turmeric-prevent-bowel-cancer

US

A Report on Curcumin's Anti-Cancer Effects by Terri Mitchell, available at **Good Health Naturally**: www.goodhealth.nu/News_Articles/050111-curcumin-anti-cancer-US.htm

Lewis Gale Hospital website. Scroll down to 'Natural and Alternative Treatments' on the main menu and click on 'Herbs and Supplements'. Then look under 'Turmeric' in the A–Z list: www.alleghanyregional.com/healthcontent.asp?page=contentselection/condensedmainindex

Memorial Sloan-Kettering Cancer Center: www.mskcc.org/mskcc/html/69401.cfm#Summary

C is for Cure

In a patient having chemotherapy or radiotherapy, a partial remission is defined as a 50% or greater decrease in the volume of a tumour. A complete remission is when all sign of the tumour has disappeared. It is tempting to see that as 'cure', but we know that many complete remissions do not last.

The situation varies from one cancer to another, but doctors begin to start talking of a cure only when there has been no sign of the cancer for five years. And, though the risk of relapse falls steadily with time, they often wait ten years before being pretty confident a tumour will not come back. Even by that strict standard, there is no doubt that many cancers are cured.

According to the most recent estimates from Cancer Research UK, half of those diagnosed with colorectal cancer in 2007 can expect to survive the disease for at least ten years. For women with breast cancer, the predicted ten-year survival rate is now 77%, which is twice what it was 30 years ago. Ten-year survival is expected to be 50% for non-Hodgkin's lymphoma, and almost 80% for the form of lymphoma known as Hodgkin's disease. The survival rate for testis cancer is 97%, and for melanoma 83%. About 75% of children with cancer survive at least five years. But, of course, there are cancers where five-year survival is still rare: it is only 6% for lung cancer, for example.

The clearest contribution to cure is made by surgery. Where a cancer is found before it has had time to spread – either close to its site of origin or to distant parts of the body – an operation can remove the problem completely. But chemotherapy and radiotherapy have also made major contributions to improved survival in cancers of the breast and testis, for example, and to the cure of blood disorders such as Hodgkin's disease and childhood leukaemia.

Sometimes, just when you think you are cured, you have only been in remission, because – guess what? – the cancer has reappeared.

I was diagnosed with breast cancer in 2002 and with inflammatory breast cancer in 2003. I was clear of tumours – in complete remission – from September 2003 to September 2005. Tumours reappeared in September 2005, and more of them in February 2006. I entered a clinical trial of the new drug lapatinib (Tykerb). Goodbye tumours. But the remission this time was short. In November 2006, they were back, and there were more of them in January 2007. So I started another new drug trial...

When I hear the words 'there is no cure for cancer', I take a long, deep look at the person who uttered them, to ascertain their agenda. Is it to reduce me to fear and despondency? Or is it merely out of ignorance? The orthodox medical profession in the United States may not use the term 'cure' because if cancer comes back, they could be sued. In the UK, I think the reluctance is more because of the outmoded idea of false hope (see 'H is for Hope (Real and False)').

TOP TIP

I do not accept that there is no cure for cancer. Live and be as well as you can be today, for who knows what tomorrow might bring.

But we do have to beware of headlines claiming this or that miracle breakthrough. Often they are talking about research that is at a very early stage. Years of work has to be done using cultures of cancer cells in the laboratory, and then animal studies, before a new drug is tried in patients. The majority of drugs that look promising in the lab fail to make it into routine clinical use either because they are not effective when faced with real cancers in real patients or because they have unexpected side effects. Even so, great progress has been made and will continue to be made – step by painstaking step.

Further information
UK

Cancer Research UK, 'Long-term survival from once-deadly cancer doubles': http://info.cancerresearchuk.org/news/archive/pressrelease/2010-07-12-deadly-cancer-survival-doubles, and 'Survival statistics for the most common cancers': http://info.cancerresearchuk.org/cancerstats/survival/latestrates

US

The Surveillance, Epidemiology and End Results (SEER) Program is the premier source for cancer statistics in the United States: http://seer.cancer.gov

For an excellent essay on cancer survival statistics, see 'The median isn't the message' by Stephen Jay Gould at CancerGuide: http://cancerguide.org/median_not_msg.html

D is for Delegation

Delegation is the art of taking the pressure off yourself by giving tasks to others.

With a diagnosis of cancer, there is much more to fit into your life. First, you deserve to have fun, and that should be at the top of the list. But a list you must have. And into the daily agenda comes a whole host of new meetings and appointments. Initially, they are diagnostic – scans, mammograms, blood tests, etc. Then comes the action plan – meetings with the surgeon, the medical oncologist, the radiation oncologist, the specialist breast care nurse, your GP or family physician, and the chemotherapy and/ or radiotherapy appointments. Get a handbag-sized notebook. Don't go anywhere without your diary. Get organized. Get a life.

You have all the usual demands on your time and energy *plus* all these extra commitments – and at a time when energy levels are less not more. This is where the art of delegation comes to the fore. If word of your diagnosis gets out among friends, family and workmates, there will undoubtedly be a plethora of phone calls, most of which will be offers of help in some way. Do not deny them – notebook out! School runs, shopping, preparation of meals... Hand over those tasks which are difficult and keep the ones that are easier (see 'F is for Friend').

Throughout all this, it is important to look your best. But instead of making the trip to the hairdresser, how about finding a hairdresser or manicurist or pedicurist – or all of the above – who will come to you? If you need to treat a friend who has saved you a complete month of school runs, what nicer way than to ask her to join you for salon therapy at home?

A team of friends arrived to winterize my garden. We had a great time and they did a great job. I treated them to a simple lunch of quiche, salad and a glass of wine. We had found a new way of having fun, and at the same time they did me a huge favour. I could have coped with the garden – it is only 30 x 20 feet and mostly paved! But it would have been onerous on my own and exhausted my energy. Plan ahead and make the most of all the love and kindness that is offered.

A B C **D** E F G H I J K L M N O P Q R S T U V W X Y Z

As an ex-stewardess on BOAC (now British Airways), I can confirm a few rules for conservation of energy (designed mainly to have enough after a flight to go partying and shopping, but the same principles apply). Do not stand when you can sit. When preparing food, or at work, or talking on the phone, make sure you are seated and in a restful pose. If you have a family or workmates, DELEGATE to THEM. They will not mind. Conserve energy to preserve energy. Under no circumstances must you allow yourself to become overtired; and, at the first sign of this, take to your bed! – along with your notebook and telephone while you think of ways and people to help you.

Allow people with cars to take you to some of your appointments. Make your appointments for a time they would be on a shopping trip near the hospital anyway. Plan ahead to minimize additional stress on yourself and to maximize contact with your friends. It is easy to abandon your friends because you only have time to communicate with your doctors. But if you do, your friends will feel left out, and you will feel isolated and alone.

TOP TIP

A diagnosis of cancer is the perfect opportunity to bathe in the light of love of family and friends, and to connect with people – don't miss out.

Further information
UK

The **CANCERactive Support Groups Directory** has a list of support groups in your area, some professionally run by a qualified therapist attached to a hospital centre, others small groups of individuals who want to help others get through these difficult times. Tel: 01280 821211. Website: www.canceractive.com

US

Lotsa Helping Hands is a private, web-based caregiving coordination service in the US that allows family, friends, neighbours and colleagues to create a community to assist a family caregiver with the daily tasks that become a challenge during times of medical crisis, caregiver exhaustion, or when caring for an elderly parent. Visit www.lotsahelpinghands.com

Each community includes an intuitive group calendar for scheduling tasks such as meals delivery and rides, a platform for securely sharing vital medical, financial and legal information with designated family members, and customizable sections for posting photos, well wishes, blogs, journals and messages.

Now when someone asks 'What can I do to help?' the answer is 'Give me your name and email address'. The system then takes over and allows people to sign up and start helping.

Reference

What Can I Do To Help? 75 Practical Ideas for Family and Friends from Cancer's Frontline by Deborah Hutton. Short Books (2005).

D is for Dental Toxins

The amalgam traditionally used for fillings was made of around 50% mercury, and there are debates as to whether this mercury can cause real problems. It could be argued that a considerable number of people are spending a lot of money on dentistry to remove mercury fillings for no reason at all. The US Food and Drug Administration, for example, concluded in 2009 that – on the available evidence – dental amalgam fillings are safe for adults and children aged six years and older. But some who have suffered from fatigue, jitteriness and visual disorders which remain unexplained by the battery of usual tests have looked at mercury as a potential cause. It is not just a case of swallowing the solid mercury in the filling – there is the vapour given off. Some say that there is not enough poisonous material in a filling to be dangerous. Others maintain that any mercury or mercury vapour entering organs such as liver, lungs, brain or kidneys is a serious toxic risk.

If you do decide to have amalgam fillings removed, it is likely – despite all precautions – that there will be a toxic onslaught on the body. So it makes sense not to have them all taken out at once and to leave lots of time for the body to recover its equilibrium between sessions.

The connection (if any) between mercury poisoning and infertility, Alzheimer's and even cancer is still being assessed. In the meantime, as someone living with cancer, I was not going to rush and have all my amalgam fillings removed. But I decided that if I had any problem with my fillings, or a metallic taste in my mouth which was not to do with the cancer drugs, I would ask my dentist to replace them with non-mercury white composite. In the full knowledge that my system could be in for a mercury pounding in the process, I would endeavour to be fit and well while undergoing treatment and take some precautionary immune boosters and vitamin C.

Mouth problems can be caused by drug treatment, and I experienced mouth sores and a sore tongue which made it difficult and painful to clean my teeth. On one of the drug trials, even my aloe vera toothpaste burned. But having a clean, healthy mouth (particularly gums) is very important for overall health and sense of well-being. I found copious use of dental floss, gentle scrubbing of teeth with no toothpaste, and a cinnamon-flavoured mouthwash did the trick. One possible factor in gum disease is the consumption of boiling hot drinks and food. If you cannot dip your finger in, it is too hot for your mouth.

TOP TIPS

Some dentists recommend taking charcoal tablets if you think you have swallowed a bit of mercury filling, along with vitamin C to help boost the immune system and the powerful antioxidant selenium.

Although there is controversy regarding the validity of claims made regarding the dangers of dental amalgams, good mouth care is important before, during and after cancer treatment. The following website offers excellent tips for mouth care during cancer treatment: http://oralhealth.deltadental.com/Adult/MedicalConditions/22,DD53.

Further information
UK

British Society for Mercury Free Dentistry, The Weathervane, 22A Moorend Park Road, Cheltenham GL53 0JY. Tel: 01242 226918. Website: www.mercuryfreedentistry.org.uk

Reference

For a sceptical view of the evidence suggesting mercury fillings cause harm, see *Skeptoid's* 'Do mercury amalgam fillings release toxic levels of mercury into the body?': http://skeptoid.com/episodes/4036.

D is for Deodorants

Aluminium salts contained in many deodorants block pores to stop perspiration. In doing so, they may find their way into the breast tissue. Parabens – chemicals used as a preservative in deodorants – have been associated with cancer. There seems to be insufficient research to confirm or refute the idea that deodorants or antiperspirants are contributing to rising rates of breast cancer. But, in 2004, researchers at the University of Reading reported that they had found parabens in breast tissue or tumour taken from cancer patients. Although small, the study concluded that underarm and breast tissues absorb these harmful chemicals through the skin. Once in the body, they can mimic the effect of oestrogen, which is known to encourage the growth of many breast cancers. The good news is that the contents of all products have to appear on the label, so it is up to us to choose what we use with care.

It may be a complete coincidence, but six months to a year before my diagnosis I had started to play tennis twice a week and had significantly stepped up my use of antiperspirants of the most chemical sort.

Cancer Research UK suggests that there is no convincing evidence that antiperspirants or deodorants cause breast cancer. But a July 2008 review by Darbre and Harvey (the Reading researchers) confirmed their continuing concern. The majority of antiperspirants and deodorants do not now contain parabens.

TOP TIP

Take the time to read the labels and beware aluminium.

Further information

UK

Breakthrough Breast Cancer charity's factsheet on deodorants and the risk of breast cancer is available from: http://breakthrough.org.uk/breast_cancer/breast_cancer_facts/risk_factors_general_information/deodorants.html

US

The **National Cancer Institute's** statement on deodorants: www.cancer.gov/cancertopics/factsheet/Risk/AP-Deo

References

What's in this Stuff? The Essential Guide to What's Really in the Products You Buy in the Supermarket by Pat Thomas. Rodale (2006).

'Concentrations of parabens in human breast tumours' by P.D. Darbre, A. Alijarrah, N.G. Coldham, M.J. Asuer and G.S. Popa. *Journal of Applied Toxicology* January–February 2004, volume 24, pages 5–13.

'Parabens esters: a review of recent studies of endocrine toxicity, absorption, esterase and human exposure, and discussion of potential human health risks' by P.D. Darbre and P.W. Harvey. *Journal of Applied Toxicology* July 2008, volume 28, pages 561–578.

D is for Depression

Depression and its companions hopelessness and despair suppress the immune system, deplete energy levels and destroy enthusiasm and positive thought – all those things which are to be encouraged in anyone, with or without cancer. On a cellular level, depression and related states are not compatible with the lean, fit fighting machine you need to be for your battle with the disease.

For someone with cancer, even being 'a bit fed up' is not an ideal state. Sometimes it is possible to shake yourself out of it by changing your environment – by doing something you really love: perhaps seeing the new James Bond movie, going ice skating or horse riding, or visiting a beautiful garden. But depression is not being 'a bit fed up'.

I remember what depression can be. Twenty years ago, I was in the middle of a divorce. I would wake in the morning, and instead of leaping into

action and off to work, I would lie in bed seeing no point in anything. I did not eat – or want to. I did not even bother to draw the curtains. And I got weaker and weaker until eventually I was found by a friend and taken to the doctor, who gave me some pills. I was very low and ended up with pneumonia. It is not a state to be taken lightly.

Real depression needs real and immediate action. The signs are tiredness; lack of energy, enthusiasm and interest in sex; poor concentration; restlessness and irritability; slowness in decision making; feelings of despair and hopelessness; and – worst scenario – not bothering to get up in the morning! Having been on the tablet route when I was 30, I believe it is important to get to the bottom of why you are depressed. It may be your diagnosis of cancer that tipped the scales. Dealing with the issues needs some expert help. The tablet is the quick fix which may get you over the first hurdle but, particularly with cancer, I like to think of the long term!

TOP TIP

Don't hold back. Depressed? Deal with it. Get help.

A diagnosis of cancer can be overwhelming. Do not consider it a sign of weakness to reach out for help. If you are having trouble dealing with the emotions you are experiencing, a mental health professional can help decide if what you are feeling is part of adjusting to the diagnosis or clinical depression or anxiety. Based on this assessment, different treatment options may be recommended. These include counselling on its own, a brief course of medication to help you through the initial difficult time, a longer course of drugs or a combination of medication and therapy. A mental health professional experienced in helping people with cancer may prove more helpful than one who has not specialized in this area.

Further information
UK

Cancer Research UK's information on coping emotionally with cancer, including fear, sadness and depression: www.cancerhelp.org.uk/coping-with-cancer/coping-emotionally

A
B
C
D
E
F
G
H
I
J
K
L
M
N
O
P
Q
R
S
T
U
V
W
X
Y
Z

US

The US **National Cancer Institute's** information on depression and cancer: www.cancer.gov/cancertopics/pdq/supportivecare/depression/Patient /page2

The **National Institute of Mental Health** brochure on depression: www. nimh.nih.gov/health/publications/depression/complete-index.shtml

For an online screening tool for depression from **PsychCentral**, see: http:// psychcentral.com/depquiz.htm

D is for Detox

Detox, or detoxification, involves eliminating from our bodies the toxins we take in from what we eat and drink and the way in which we live in our increasingly polluted world. An added benefit is that detox is usually accompanied by weight loss, because of the list of banned items. Booze is generally completely off limits, as are chocolates, refined sugars and caffeine. So a detox diet can make you feel quite unwell as you 'come down' from your own particular 'fix'. It is not until after the detox that you really reap the benefits: more energy, in a calm and focused way, and the knowledge that your system is in its best fighting form.

Detox's companion is De-stress. This can relate to stress as in 'immune overload' or stress as in anxiety. When detoxing do not be surprised if you feel emotional. While you might consider it a physical process, there is no doubt that detoxing has effects at a mental and emotional level.

There are various ways of detoxing. These range from a juice and water fast, a gentle detox diet, to a much more ferocious regime including colonic irrigation or hydrotherapy (see 'C is for Colonic Irrigation (or Colonic Hydrotherapy)'). Detoxification plays a major role in any alternative approach to fighting cancer. The theory is that removing toxins enables the body to regain its natural energy flow and so restores the immune system to peak performance. In the alternative approach, diet and nutrition are part of integrating body, mind and spirit. But detoxing should be equally valuable as a complement to orthodox treatment.

If not actually adding to its efficacy, it will certainly help you tolerate it more easily.

Further information
References

The Seven-Day Total Cleanse: A Revolutionary New Juice Fast and Yoga Plan to Purify Your Body and Clarify the Mind by Mary Mcguire-Wien. McGraw-Hill (2009).

Juice Fasting and Detoxification: Use the Healing Power of Fresh Juice to Feel Young and Look Great. The Fastest Way to Restore Your Health by Steve Meyerowitz. Book Publishing Company, 6th edition (1999).

The New Detox Diet by Elson Haas. Celestial Arts (2004).

D is for D-glucarate

We are increasingly aware of the effect of harmful chemicals on our health and our environment, tobacco tar still being top of the list of carcinogens from which we are most at risk. There is also concern about hormones and hormone-like chemicals and their link to the development of breast cancer and possibly other cancers too.

In the body, the process of glucuronidation is one means by which circulating toxins are bound and then eliminated via the liver. Hormones such as oestrogen, produced naturally in the body, may also be removed in this way. Normally, glucuronidation works efficiently, but it is possible that the system could be overloaded by toxins, leading to their reabsorption rather than excretion.

The enzyme beta-glucuronidase inhibits glucuronidation but can itself be inhibited by calcium D-glucarate. This dietary supplement is a version of the glucaric acid found in many common vegetables such as broccoli, which some regard as 'superfoods' for their antioxidant and immune-boosting qualities. Other natural sources include cabbage, brussels sprouts, cauliflower (like broccoli, members of the brassica family) and alfalfa, as well as grapefruits, apples, oranges, cherries and apricots.

There are studies in animals suggesting that D-glucarate can increase excretion of oestrogen and carcinogens, including compounds found in cigarette smoke. There is also some laboratory evidence that it can inhibit certain of the stages involved in the development and growth of cancers. We do not yet have evidence that this is the case in people. It could be argued that taking a D-glucarate supplement is reasonable in times of stress or illness. But, if you are taking any prescription medication, please consult your physician or pharmacist. Calcium D-glucarate could affect the way the body metabolizes and excretes many drugs (especially hormones) and so might reduce their effectiveness.

TOP TIP

Eat your greens! Consider taking this supplement to boost your body's defences! But first please check this product's suitability with your doctor.

Further information
UK
> **The Institute for Optimum Nutrition**: www.ion.ac.uk

US
> **Memorial Sloan-Kettering Cancer Center**: www.mskcc.org/mskcc/html/ 69158.cfm

> **WebMD** information: www.webmd.com/vitamins-supplements/ingredient mono-136-CALCIUM+D-GLUCARATE.aspx?activeIngredientId=136& activeIngredientName=CALCIUM+D-GLUCARATE&source=3

Reference
> *D-Glucarate: A Nutrient Against Cancer* by Thomas J. Slaga PhD and Judi Quilici-Timmcke MS. McGraw-Hill Contemporary (2000).

D is for Diagnosis

At the age of 48 and a half, it did not occur to me that the large egg-shaped lump high in my right breast was anything other than a strained pectoral muscle. Over the previous few months I had been lifting some heavy paving stones and then had been sailing. In any event, the lump was nothing like the 'pea' or 'bean' I associated with breast cancer.

I had just finished supervizing a major project and was a little run down with a nasty cold. I did not want anything to spoil my few days lapping up the last of the summer sun with friends in the south of France. So I paid a quick visit to my GP to see if I should take some antibiotics with me, in case the cold developed into a chest infection. He asked me various questions. I did not think to mention the lump, but I did mention the rather sore lymph node under my arm. He cross-questioned me about checking my breasts regularly and said in passing that malignant lumps are not always the size of peas or beans – they can resemble more a hard-boiled egg. He was keen to examine me there and then, but I was keen to leave. So I made an excuse, said I'd be back to see him on my return and escaped.

We played five hours of tennis a day, after which none of us had much energy for partying, so we had dinner and early nights. My cold disappeared and I was beginning to feel really fit and well. Changing one night, I asked my husband to run his fingers over my 'strained muscle'. He was in no doubt and described it as a 'lump'. On the Sunday, our husbands had to return home, leaving my friend and me to have one further day of shopping and tennis. This time was almost a preparation in mind, body and soul for what was to come.

I didn't really mention my lump to my friend B until we were taxiing along the runway. But B leaped into action as we drove into central London. We made phone calls and I telephoned my long-suffering GP. This was Tuesday. I was booked to see a specialist at 8.30 on Thursday morning.

Thursday 26 September. At 8.30 a.m., my husband and I arrive at the Royal Marsden Hospital to see the surgeon, who is reassuringly brusque. Pretty immediately I am on the examination table having an ultrasound scan. Ultrasound jelly was placed over the breast and a pencil-like sensor traced over the skin. It is not even a remotely unpleasant experience. Ultrasound waves bouncing back from any surfaces they meet create a picture on the monitor screen. We can both see the lump. It is a clean lump, like a small cherry nut. The sides do not have tendril-like growth, and this is deemed to be positive. Also, viewed from the other side there is a clear line, but with a small node on top.

A
B
C
D
E
F
G
H
I
J
K
L
M
N
O
P
Q
R
S
T
U
V
W
X
Y
Z

I ask whether, in the consultant's experience, this looks like a benign lump. He thinks not. I ask how he can possibly tell, and he says it's because he has seen hundreds before. But to be sure whether there are cancer cells present, I must have a needle biopsy. The surgeon anaesthetizes the area. Then – remarkably quickly, because I am thinking it takes time for the local anaesthetic to take effect – there is the biopsy needle. Still lying on the examination table, I look towards the screen to see if I can see the needle inserted into the lump, but the monitor has been turned off. There is no associated pain or discomfort.

Anyone who has had to wait for test results knows how waiting can almost be worse than the worst possible result. I devised a strategy for keeping busy: never had the house been cleaner, with all the cupboards turned out. It is important to keep in a positive state of mind – so if cupboard clearing is not the solution for you, see a film or do something that you have always wanted to do. Breathing techniques, yoga and pilates may also help. Once that negative inner voice has a chance to be heard, worry and anxiety insidiously creep into your mind.

When the biopsy results came through and I was told I had cancer, I could think of nothing to say except 'Are you sure?' Disbelief was followed by total shock. This was not denial but rather a sense of 'this is it, my life is about to end'. In retrospect, why on earth should I think that? I was not lying in hospital having been blown up by a bomb. It was a totally irrational mindset. I stood there having just returned from a long weekend of tennis coaching for five hours a day. I was a bit tired, but very fit. Obviously, cancer is a life-threatening disease. But I wish someone had said, 'Your life is threatened but you are OK now and likely to be fine. You need to look at your diet and lifestyle. Be as well as you can, by whatever means you can.' As it was, I stood there like a rabbit in the headlights.

Early symptoms can be misleading – I thought my problem was a strained muscle. (There is also the possibility, of course, that I was trying to ignore it in the hope it would just go away.) I cannot stress enough how important it is to be aware of your body. If you notice or feel any changes, *go to your doctor immediately.* The smaller the lump – whether it be in the breast, the prostate or anywhere else – the easier it is to deal with. Even if it is cancerous, you may get away without chemotherapy or radiation if a surgeon can remove the lump and leave margins clear of cancer.

TOP TIP

Would you share a cab with a terrorist? Well, a cancer cell is a terrorist in hiding – a potentially aggressive threat to your life, not your new best friend! Get checked!

Further information
UK

Cancer Research UK on the importance of early diagnosis: http:// info.cancerresearchuk.org/spotcancerearly/cancersignandsymptoms/ whyisearlydiagnosisimportant/index.htm

US

American Cancer Society guidelines for the early detection of cancer: www.cancer.org/Healthy/FindCancerEarly/CancerScreeningGuidelines/ american-cancer-society-guidelines-for-the-early-detection-of-cancer

D is for Diet and Nutritional Therapy (or Food, Glorious Food)

It never ceases to amaze me that the link between cancer and food is not a universally accepted fact and, as such, one of the first considerations of someone affected by cancer, or at high risk and trying to prevent it. Following hundreds of studies involving many thousands of people, experts believe that around 30% of cancers occurring in the Western world relate to aspects of our diet such as our high intake of processed foods and animal fats and our relatively low intake of fresh fruit and vegetables. But, despite the evidence, there are still people who do not accept that diet and cancer are linked. How can they not be related? The real issue is the *degree* to which diet is a contributory factor, and how much it contributes to different kinds of cancer. One major research paper (published in 2003) combined the results from almost 50 studies including in total more than half a million women. It found that those eating large amounts of saturated fat – in meat, cheese and other full-fat dairy products – were 20% more likely to develop breast cancer. That is a clear enough message to reduce intake of such foods, and to increase fruit and veg. Recently, financial necessity has been leading more people to grow their own and to exercise their own quality control. This can only be positive.

Any holistic approach recognizes the importance of the food that we eat and the potential damage – poisoning at worst, unnecessary stress on the system at best – if we do not take care in this regard. We need only think of mad cow disease (variant CJD), of farm animals injected with high levels of antibiotics, and of battery chickens fed we are not sure what and never seeing the light of day. Living with cancer means asking the right questions about what we eat, about how it is grown (has it been sprayed with pesticides?) or what it has been fed. On the positive side, living with cancer means making sure you are getting the vitamins and minerals you need (see 'A is for Antioxidant Vitamins and Minerals'; 'V is for Vitamins').

Eating the right things provides the body with a balanced diet and all the minerals, trace elements, vitamins and proteins needed to maintain its most effective condition. The aim of nutritional therapy in cancer care is to support patients through their orthodox medical treatment and enable them to feel as well as possible. This can be done by helping them tolerate drug regimes better through minimizing side effects, by reducing the risk of infection through supporting the immune system before, during and after treatment, and by maintaining a steady weight and avoiding weight loss. Nutritional therapy may well have a role after treatment also, reducing the possibility of recurrence by a strict regime of nutritional care. Nutritional therapies range from the radical, such as is advocated by Gerson (see 'G is for Gerson Therapy'), to more general healthy-eating approaches such as the Plant Programme (see 'References' on page 122).

If you already have cancer, the dilemma is which of the wide range of nutritional therapies one should try. There is a mind-boggling array of books on the subject of the cancer diet, and different cancers may require different diets. But most recommend avoiding large amounts of sugar, fat and alcohol, so weight loss is likely. The paradox is that we fear the weight loss, commonly described as 'wasting away', that is associated with advanced cancer. So when you are weighed in for treatment, finding no loss of weight is generally regarded as positive, and there is delight in an increased weight of a pound or two. Apart from eating the right foods, the other main criterion is to avoid toxins (see 'C is for Chemicals').

There is a general strategy, and there are certain specific things that I found really made a difference. For example, I am convinced that the intravenous vitamin C injection prior to a ten-hour surgical procedure helped hugely with how I felt after the operation and my speedy recuperation. I also had homeopathic support to rid myself of the after-effects of the anaesthetic, and arginine and arnica to aid healing.

During chemotherapy, I had a regime of antioxidants, vitamins, immune support and fish oil in capsule form. I did not miss a single treatment and felt as well as one can with no hair, eyebrows and eyelashes! I did also avoid many things I love – chocolates, coffee, wine...

With a mouthful of sweet teeth and a craving for chocolate, sugar was a large part of my diet in the past. I find ANY type of diet difficult to stick to, particularly the nut and seed-loaf type. But through my treatment I did manage not to eat red meat and I replaced dairy with soya or rice milk.

Just a few reminders about what lucky people can eat in order to build up their strength and *not* resort to junk food! The suggestions refer to organic foods. In recipes including wheat and dairy products, substitutes can be found in rice flour and soya milk.

❧ Breakfast ❧
Bowl of cereal with banana
Eggs, lean bacon, sausage, tomato, mushrooms and fried
wholemeal bread
Pancakes with maple syrup
Smoked haddock with a poached egg and
slices of wholemeal toast

☙ Lunch ❧
Jacket potato with filling
– tuna and sweetcorn
– organic melted cheese and tomato
– with ham and the above
Omelette – cheese/ham/tomato

☙ Dinner ❧
Chicken and ham pie
Steak and kidney pie
Pasta

☙ Snacks/desserts ❧
Smoothies with soya ice cream
The dessert trolley is yours!

Liz Butler, Senior Nutritional Therapist, Penny Brohn Cancer Care (formerly Bristol Cancer Help Centre), suggests the alternative menu below in line with their Bristol Approach to Healthy Eating – a set of guidelines designed to support the general health and well-being of those with cancer.

☙ Breakfast ❧
Oat porridge
Muesli
A selection of breads and toast
A selection of spreads (e.g. fruit spreads and nut butters)
Fresh and dried fruit
Hot option – poached egg, grilled mushrooms, tomatoes and baked beans

☙ Snack ❧
Beetroot, carrot and apple juice

☙ Lunch ❧
Lentil and tomato soup
Lemon and tarragon chicken or sweet potato and tofu rosti

Salad selection
Fresh fruit

⌒ **Snack** ⌒
Date and walnut flapjack

⌒ **Dinner** ⌒
Vegetable tagine with rice
Fresh fruit

TOP TIP

Buy organic – this is likely to cost more, but there are other ways of economizing. If you think your diet might lack beneficial vitamins, cheat – take supplements (but check with your doctor first).

A nutritional therapist should be an integral part of the cancer team. What is required is an initial assessment, a dietary programme to help you through treatment, and a post-treatment plan to reach and maintain optimum health.

Further information
UK

British Association of Nutritional Therapists Tel: 08706 061284. Website: www.bant.org.uk

Macmillan Cancer Support's information on the 'Building-up diet', designed to help slow down or stop further weight loss due to cancer or its treatments. Website: www.macmillan.org.uk/Cancerinformation/ Livingwithandaftercancer/Eatingwell

See **Penny Brohn Cancer Care's** evidence-based information sheet on nutrition. *The Bristol Approach to Healthy Eating: A guide on how to maintain optimal nutrient levels whilst living with cancer* is downloadable from www. pennybrohncancercare.org. (These new nutritional guidelines, published in 2010, form part of the Bristol Approach used by Penny Brohn Cancer Care and are now being adopted within the National Health Service as advice for people living with cancer to help manage their own long-term condition.)

The Bristol Approach 7 Day Recipe Plan by Elizabeth Butler, Senior Nutritional Therapist, and Anna Ralph, Head Chef, Penny Brohn Cancer Care (2010) is also downloadable from www.pennybrohncancercare.org

World Cancer Research Fund UK's booklet *Eating Well and Being Active Following Cancer Treatment* is downloadable from their website: www.wcrf-uk. org/PDFs/Eating_Well_for_Cancer_Prevention.pdf

US

National Cancer Institute's eating hints for before, during and after cancer treatment: www.cancer.gov/cancertopics/coping/eatinghints

Centers for Disease Control and Prevention guidelines for a healthy diet: www.fruitsandveggiesmatter.gov

The **American Cancer Society** has excellent information for cancer patients with separate sections for before, during and after treatment (two links are provided, but scout around the site as there are other pages of interest):

1. Nutrition and exercise guidelines from the **National Cancer Institute**: www.cancer.org/Healthy/EatHealthyGetActive/ACSGuidelineson NutritionPhysicalActivityforCancerPrevention/index?sitearea=PED

2. More specific information on diets that may be recommended to cancer patients: www.cancer.org/Treatment/TreatmentsandSideEffects/Comple mentaryandAlternativeMedicine/DietandNutrition/index?sitearea=ETO

Brett Moore's top twelve fruits and vegetables you should buy organically grown: http://gourmetfood.about.com/od/slowfoodorganiclocal/a/organicproduce. htm

References

Anticancer: A New Way of Life by David Servan-Schreiber. Michael Joseph (2008).

The Rainbow Diet by Chris Woolhams. Health Issues Ltd (2008).

Your Life in Your Hands: Understand, Prevent and Overcome Breast Cancer and Ovarian Cancer by Jane Plant. Virgin Books (2007).

Foods to Fight Cancer: Essential Foods to Help Prevent Cancer by Richard Béliveau and Denis Gingras. Dorling Kindersley (2007).

The Plant Programme: Recipes for Fighting Breast and Prostate Cancer by Jane Plant and Gill Tidey. Virgin Books (2004).

Nutrition and Cancer: State-of-the-Art by Sandra Goodman, Health Research Ltd (2003); order from www.drsgoodman.com/books-goodman.

Breast Cancer: Beyond Convention: The World's Foremost Authorities on Complementary and Alternative Medicine Offer Advice on Healing edited by Mary Tagliferri, Isaac Cohen and Debu Tripathy. James Bennett Ltd (2002).

'Diet, nutrition and the prevention of cancer' by Timothy Key and colleagues. *Public Health Nutrition* 2004, volume 7, pages 187–200.

D is for Drugs (Targeted Drugs)

See also 'C is for Chemotherapy'

A cell that becomes malignant gives rise to a cancer because several abnormal things happen. Typically, the cell starts a process of uncontrolled division: it reproduces itself far more frequently than the body requires for the purposes of repair and replacement. Second, malignant cells do not die when they should: their severe abnormality would normally activate self-destruct mechanisms (termed apoptosis), but these fail to operate. Third, the huddle of abnormal cells begins to secrete molecules that cause neighbouring normal cells to form the blood vessels that will bring the cancer the oxygen and nutrients it requires for further rapid growth. The abnormal cells also produce substances that break down the barriers formed by healthy cells, allowing the cancer to spread into surrounding tissues.

So we have a range of problems: the uncontrolled proliferation of abnormal cells, their failure to commit suicide, the formation of new blood vessels (called angiogenesis) which will sustain the tumour in its growth, and the invasion by the cancer of healthy tissue. All of these processes are controlled by specific molecules, and each of these cancer-promoting molecules can be a target for anti-cancer drugs.

Such targeted agents have ushered in a new era of therapy which is far more sophisticated than we have previously had. It offers far more options and can be tailored to the circumstances of individual patients in a way never before possible. The aim of a chemotherapy drug is simply to kill quickly dividing cells. These drugs cannot distinguish between good cells that divide rapidly because of their healthy function, such as those producing hair, and bad cells that divide rapidly because they are cancerous. (This is why chemo patients may lose their hair.) Targeted anti-cancer drugs on the other hand seek to block the abnormal growth-promoting signals that are found *only* within or around cancer cells. At the moment, they do this imperfectly. So targeted drugs too have side effects. But they are different from those found with chemotherapy, and targeted drugs in general cause fewer and less severe problems.

How targeted drugs work

Receptors on the cell are like docking stations for molecules (growth factors) circulating in the blood. When a growth factor activates a receptor, a growth promoting signal is sent to the cell nucleus, 1.

Drugs can prevent this happening in several different ways. Sites at which targeted drugs act are shown as 2-4.

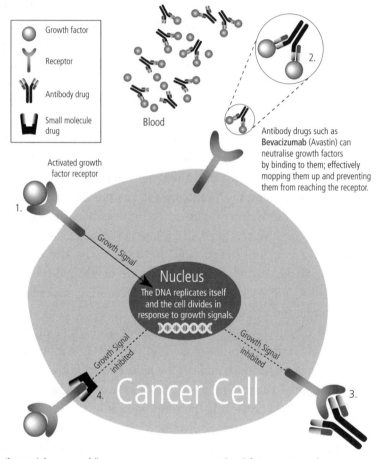

Growth factor

Receptor

Antibody drug

Small molecule drug

Blood

Activated growth factor receptor

1.

Antibody drugs such as **Bevacizumab** (Avastin) can neutralise growth factors by binding to them; effectively mopping them up and preventing them from reaching the receptor.

Growth Signal

Nucleus
The DNA replicates itself and the cell divides in response to growth signals.

Growth Signal Inhibited

Growth Signal Inhibited

4.

3.

Cancer Cell

Even if a growth factor successfully attaches to the part of the receptor outside the cell, small molecule drugs can bind to the internal portion of the receptor and prevent it from sending the growth signal. Examples include the drugs **Erlotinib** (Tarceva) and **Gefitinib** (Iressa).

Growth factor receptors can be blocked by drugs that attach to but do not activate them. **Trastuzamab** (Herceptin) is an example of a drug that acts in this way, like a key which fits a lock but cannot open the door.

How targeted drugs work

Even if an activated receptor starts to send a growth signal to the nucleus, the message can still be stopped by small molecule drugs that block stations along its route (5a-c).

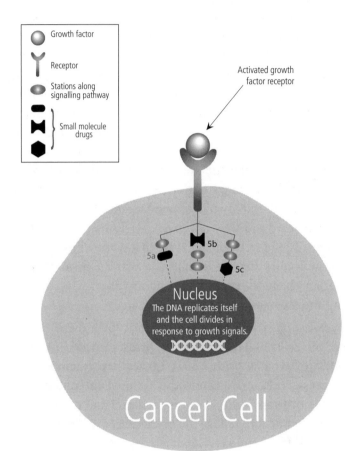

There are several stages along a signalling pathway, and drugs can block the pathway at different points. The problem is that - as with a passenger on the London Underground rail system, or the New York subway - a signal can take alternative routes to its destination if its usual path is blocked. So it may be necessary to use drugs that block several pathways at once (5a, 5b and 5c). Devising combinations of targeted agents that achieve this is now the big challenge for cancer specialists.

A
B
C
D
E
F
G
H
I
J
K
L
M
N
O
P
Q
R
S
T
U
V
W
X
Y
Z

The 'abs' and the 'ibs'

We have talked about the different cancer-related processes that can be targeted with drugs. We can also distinguish between the different *ways* these new drugs act.

Certain drugs seek to 'mop up' growth factors circulating in the blood before they get a chance to bind to and activate growth receptors on cells. Other drugs prevent growth factors gaining access to receptors by occupying them themselves (acting like a key that fits in the lock but does not open the door). Then there are drugs that work within the cancer cell itself to block the transmission of messages from an activated growth receptor to the cell nucleus where the command to divide is put into effect.

Drugs that act outside the cell or on its surface are often large molecule monoclonal antibodies based on genetically engineered bits of our own immune system. Their chemical names end in 'ab', and they are given by slow infusion into a vein at intervals of a week or so. Drugs that work within the cell are small molecules and are usually taken in the form of daily tablets. Their chemical names often end in 'ib'.

Among the most important now in use are:

- *Trastuzumab (Herceptin)* targets a receptor for growth signals found on cells in HER2-positive breast cancers. (Around 20–30% of women with breast cancer have tumours that overexpress HER2.) Herceptin can be used in combination with chemotherapy drugs such as paclitaxel and docetaxel in adjuvant treatment to reduce the risk a cancer will return after surgery, and to extend survival when the disease is advanced. There is a risk of side effects on the heart, so Herceptin may not be appropriate in someone with a history of cardiovascular problems.

- *Bevacizumab (Avastin)* disrupts the ability of a tumour to create new blood vessels – it is an anti-angiogenic drug. Since developing blood vessels is something all cancers must do if they are to grow beyond a certain size, Avastin is effective in a range of tumour types. It was first shown to extend survival (when used in combination with chemotherapy) in bowel cancer, but works also in kidney cancer, certain forms of lung cancer, and in cancer of the breast. High blood pressure is a relatively common side effect, as is skin rash. This antibody works by neutralizing a natural protein called vascular endothelial growth factor.

- *Cetuximab (Erbitux)* attaches itself to (and so blocks) a cell surface receptor for epidermal growth factor. It is used alone or in combination with the chemotherapy drug irinotecan to treat bowel cancer that has recurred, and, along with radiotherapy, in head and neck cancer. Common side effects include tiredness and rash.

- *Rituximab (Mabthera)* is an antibody that homes in on a protein found on the surface of certain white cells which become cancerous in non-Hodgkin's lymphoma. Frequently given in combination with chemotherapy, it can cause flu-like symptoms, low blood pressure, rash and anaemia.

- *Imatinib (Glivec or Gleevec)* is a small molecule with a big place in the history of cancer treatment. A particular form of leukemia called CML occurs when parts of two chromosomes become switched. Cells with this abnormality produce a protein which causes them to grow out of control. Imatinib was designed specifically to target this molecule and has proved enormously successful in extending by many years the lives of people with CML. Diarrhoea is a common side effect but can be relatively easily controlled.

- *Sunitinib (Sutent), sorafenib (Nexavar) and pazopanib (Votrient)* are beneficial in the most common form of kidney cancer. They are used when the tumour has spread and work by reducing the growth rate of cancer cells and by inhibiting formation of new blood vessels. Sorafenib is also helpful in cancer of the liver. Side effects include tiredness and soreness of the palms and soles of the feet. Pazopanib is approved in the USA and Europe but may not be available in the UK under the National Health Service.

- *Erlotinib (Tarceva) and gefitinib (Iressa)* are used to treat certain forms of advanced lung cancer. These drugs prevent the growth signal being transmitted from the epidermal growth factor receptor on the surface of the cell to the cell nucleus. Frequent side effects include rash and diarrhoea.

A B C D E F G H I J K L M N O P Q R S T U V W X Y Z

- *Lapatinib (Tyverb or Tykerb)* can be used to slow the growth of HER2-positive breast cancers which have stopped responding to trastuzumab. It is not available in the UK on the National Health Service.

The general pattern is for a new drug to be assessed first in one form of cancer, in which there is particular reason for thinking it might work. Success in one tumour type is then followed by clinical trials in another. This process is expensive, and the cost of targeted drugs is high (so health providers face a major challenge in making them available to all who stand to benefit). The process is also often frustratingly slow. But progress is clearly being made.

TOP TIP

There will never be a drug that cures all people of all cancers. Cancer is many different diseases. Even within a specific organ, such as the lung, there are many types of tumour. The lung has several kinds of cells, and each kind has its own form of cancer. Within each type of cell, there is a range of different genetic abnormalities that can cause uncontrolled growth. Each will require a tailored treatment. That is the extent of the problem. On the other hand, we now have the understanding and the tools to develop drugs that will do the very specific things that are needed.

Distrust headlines about breakthrough cures: the process is piecemeal and slow, but we are making progress even with cancers like melanoma which have always been very difficult to treat. Take encouragement from our experience with treating AIDS. True, when compared with a cancer cell, the virus responsible for AIDS is relatively simple. When drug developers were told the weak points of the virus, they said, 'Give us ten years, and we'll sort it out.' In less than that time, they had produced drugs that turned otherwise deadly HIV infection into a disease that people can live with for decades. That is probably what will happen with the common cancers, but it will take a while.

E is for Echinacea

Echinacea preparations (made from the North American coneflower) are among the most popular complementary therapies. They are widely thought to serve as a stimulant for the body's immune system by increasing the number and activity of cells which fight invading organisms such as bacteria and viruses. Any increased resistance to infection is potentially useful for patients with cancer, especially if they are undergoing a treatment like chemotherapy which damages the immune system.

There is reasonably good evidence that echinacea preparations are effective in treating the common cold if taken soon after infection with the virus. Evidence that echinacea helps prevent colds is less consistent, and the effects of taking the herb for long periods are uncertain. Beneficial effects on cells that can fight tumour cells and on wound healing have been suggested.

Echinacea products vary greatly in the proportion of plant flower, stem and root used in their manufacture, in the way that the plant material is extracted, and even in the species of coneflower used. But there is considerable scientific interest in assessing the mechanism of action and effects of standardized preparations of the plant and in isolating its active chemical components.

Further information

UK

Cancer Research UK: www.cancerhelp.org.uk/about-cancer/treatment/complementary-alternative/therapies/echinacea

US

Memorial Sloan-Kettering Cancer Center: www.mskcc.org/mskcc/html/69209.cfm

ConsumerLab have tested a number of echinacea supplements in the US: www.consumerlab.com/reviews/echinacea_review/echinacea. It is not possible to include the entire list of approved products but **GNC** Herbal Plus Standardized Echinacea Extract and **Nature's Bounty** Natural Whole Herb Echinacea are readily available.

References

'Results of five randomized studies of the immunomodulatory activity of preparations of Echinacea' by D. Melchart and colleagues. *Journal of Alternative and Complementary Medicine* 1995, volume 1, pages 145–160.

'Herbal medicines and perioperative care' by M. Ang-Lee and colleagues, *Journal of the American Medical Association* 2001, volume 286, pages 208–216.

'Echinacea for preventing and treating the common cold' by K. Linde and colleagues. *Cochrane Database Systematic Reviews* January 2006.

'Evaluation of Echinacea for the prevention and treatment of the common cold' by S.A. Shah and colleagues. *Lancet Infectious Disease* 2007, volume 7, pages 473–480.

E is for EEG Neurofeedback

See 'B is for Brainwave Therapy'

E is for Emotions

Be prepared for the emotional rollercoaster of your life – for this is exactly what it may be.

Fear is probably the first emotion upon diagnosis. But remember you are not alone. One in three people will have a cancer diagnosed at some time in their lives.

Then comes anger. Many feel 'Why me?' And if you are not angry about that, there is bound to be at least one aspect of your care that drives you to justifiable fury.

Several of my medical team are true heroes whom I would have been unlikely to meet without the diagnosis of cancer. These people were with me through the difficult times and loved any excuse to celebrate victory, no matter how small. But not all my experiences were good.

Once, having arrived at the chemo department at 8.00 a.m. as instructed, I was kept waiting to be seen by a registrar. Several hours later, he saw fit to go out for lunch while I was still sitting there. I was then told I was too late to have my chemo that day and should come back tomorrow. I was just about to explode when my oncologist came in and authorized it himself at 4.00 p.m.

The potential for feeling you could scream the place down or weep for England is huge, so be prepared. Do not leave your sense of humour behind. You will need it.

A huge amount of all this goes on in the waiting room. It is ridiculous, given the above, to think that there is any possibility of calm. But if you are reading this book in the waiting room, turn quickly to 'B is for Breath and Breathing' and practise the exercises.

Take care – some think that cells reflect, monitor and store emotions. This is absolutely fine if they are positive emotions, but not if they are negative.

TOP TIP
Smile, God loves you.

Further information
UK

Cancer Research UK: www.cancerhelp.org.uk/coping-with-cancer/coping-emotionally

US

American Cancer Association: www.cancer.org/Treatment/TreatmentsandSideEffects/EmotionalSideEffects/CopingwithCancerinEverydayLife/index

The **Mayo Clinic** discussion on emotions and cancer: www.mayoclinic.com/health/cancer-survivor/CA00071

References

The Human Side of Cancer by Jimmie C. Holland MD, of Memorial Sloan-Kettering Cancer Center, explores the broad range of emotions people with cancer and their loved ones experience from diagnosis through treatment and its aftermath. The first two chapters are available online at: www.humansideofcancer.com/default.htm.

Wendy Harpham is both a physician and cancer survivor. She has written several books and all are recommended. *Happiness in a Storm: Facing Illness and Embracing Life as a Healthy Survivor* is an excellent discussion on living well with cancer. Links to Dr Harpham's publications: http://wendyharpham.com/pages/publications.htm.

The Biology of Belief: Unleashing the Power of Consciousness, Matter and Miracles by Bruce H. Lipton. Hay House UK (2008).

Molecules of Emotion: Why You Feel the Way You Feel by Candace Pert. Pocket Books (1999).

A B C D E F G H I J K L M N O P Q R S T U V W X Y Z

E is for Energy

I do not mean the quick fix of a Mars bar to help you work, rest and play. Neither do I mean absence of tiredness or fatigue. I mean energy in the cosmic sense.

A while back, a friend came round for tea. I had been feeling lethargic and fed up because of lack of progress with this book. I was not lacking enthusiasm, just energy. Instead of sitting in the largest room in the house, we sat in my tiny study round the fire, surrounded by my books and papers all over the floor. We talked about girlie things, hair highlights, diet and exercise, but I was conscious of something somehow changing in the room. After we said goodbye, I returned to my study, sat at my desk and started to write. Apart from a quick helping of Chinese takeaway at about 8.00 p.m. I continued until 3 o'clock in the morning, focused and energetically. How might this be explained? Was there some other form of communication going on while we friends chattered? Did I feel my friend's support and strength on some other level, which then inspired me? She came round for tea and brought me a present of some great energy.

The explanation fits neatly into a concept of quantum physics referred to as Zero Point Field. Energy consists of particles and molecules which are never at rest: they are always in a state of motion. We are energy and live in a field or sea of energy with everything connected to every other thing in the world like an invisible web. Particles and molecules resonate or fluctuate and this can be detected even at temperatures of absolute zero. My friend had come into my working space resonating with positive vibrations. As she is quite religious, she may even have said a prayer to give me strength and get me back on track with my writing, which we hope will help others. And, hey presto – energy changed in the room and in me.

Take this explanation from quantum physics and turn now to healing. Is this why a cancer patient is advised to beware of negative forces and to have a positive attitude? Because, for some unexplained reason, patients with a positive attitude tend to survive, or at least survive longer. Or have we the hint of a far greater truth – that molecules and particles in motion are always exchanging information?

It has been suggested that we are all surrounded by a huge force field of dynamic energy that we can 'tap' into. But most of us do not – because we are on the run, we do not understand it and do not know how to. An energy healer, such as a Reiki or spiritual healer, facilitates our ability to tap into this source of universal energy. It is almost like radio wavelengths: there are different frequencies, and you need to be taught how to tune in!

There is an idea that energy healing uses a map of consciousness called the Human Energy Field to trace symptoms to their causes. Perhaps this relates to chakras or auras. If one has an emotional 'block' when dealing with something difficult such as divorce, bereavement or a diagnosis of cancer, the energy does not flow easily. This causes an imbalance in the energy field and can lead to tension and ill health as communication on a cellular level becomes disturbed. Clearing the energy field helps to repair this and improve well-being.

Energy healing techniques include chakra balancing, colour healing, sound healing, past-life regression, emotional clearing, and clearing ancestral patterns. Guidance is also given on a healthy, natural lifestyle including diet, detoxification and exercise, along with coaching on how to manage your energy in daily life.

TOP TIP

May the force be with you!

Further information

References

Women's Bodies, Women's Wisdom: The Complete Guide to Women's Health and Wellbeing by Christiane Northrup. Piatkus (2009); especially Chapter 4, 'The Female Energy System'.

The Healer's Manual: A Beginner's Guide To Energy Therapies by Ted Andrews. Llewellyn Publications (2002).

Defy Gravity: Healing Beyond the Boundaries of Ordinary Reason by Caroline Myss. Hay House UK (2009).

The Field: The Quest for the Secret Force of the Universe by Lynne McTaggart. Element Thorsons (2003).

Quantum Healing: Exploring The Frontiers of Mind/Body Medicine by Deepak Chopra. Bantam (1989).

E is for Essiac

Essiac is a herbal remedy, originally used by the Ojibwa tribe of Canadian First Nations, that is said to cleanse the blood and promote cell repair. The main medicinal herbs which it contains are rhubarb root, sheep sorrel, slippery elm inner bark and burdock root. It is claimed that combining these four herbs produces an additional synergy.

The benefits of Essiac were discovered by Nurse Rene Caisse who died in 1978 having sold the rights for the remedy to Resperin in Canada. The company believes that Essiac can help purge toxic build-up of waste from the body, that it is rich in essential vitamins and minerals which help strengthen cells, and that it is without adverse effects.

There is no claim that Essiac is an alternative to orthodox cancer treatment but there are anecdotal stories of people being helped. Cancer Research UK says that there is no scientific evidence Essiac can cure cancer and also lists possible side effects.

TOP TIP

It is important to buy from a reliable source to avoid counterfeits. I find Essiac tea completely undrinkable, as indeed I find most herbal teas. Luckily, Essiac is also available as a herbal tincture.

Further information
UK

Cancer Research UK: www.cancerhelp.org.uk/about-cancer/treatment/complementary-alternative/therapies/Essiac

US

The US **National Cancer Institute** on Essiac: www.cancer.gov/cancerinfo/pdq/cam/Essiac

Reference

Essiac: The Secrets of Rene Caisse's Herbal Pharmacy by Sheila Snow and Mali Klein. Newleaf (2001).

E is for Exceptional or Expert Patient

The term 'exceptional patient' is used by Bernie Siegel – a distinguished American surgeon with a wealth of experience of cancer and cancer patients (see 'Reference' on the following page). He says, 'Physicians must realize that the patients they consider difficult or uncooperative are those who are most likely to get well.' He continues, 'Exceptional patients refuse to be victims.' That means not just victims of the disease but also victims of an arrogant doctor who will not answer questions, or of a dismissive oncologist, or an unsympathetic nurse. 'Exceptional patients manifest the will to live in its most potent form. They take charge of their lives... And they work hard to achieve health and peace of mind. They do not rely on doctors to take the initiative but rather use them as members of a team, demanding the utmost in technique, resourcefulness, concern, and open-mindedness. If they're not satisfied, they change doctors.'

People respond very differently to a diagnosis of cancer. There are those who want the doctor to tell them what to do so that it can all be over and done with as quickly as possible. Others want to engage in battle. They see knowledge as power. They want answers and they want to know the options. These are the patients who have surfed the web and may sometimes have found out more about new treatments than their doctors. At the very least, they will know enough to ask the right questions.

As Bernie Siegel says, 'Exceptional patients do not abandon hope. Even if what you most hope for – a complete cure – doesn't come to pass, the hope itself can sustain you to accomplish many things in the meantime. Refusal to hope is nothing more than a decision to die.'

TOP TIP

Exceptional patients recognize that there are silver linings to seemingly black clouds.

Further information
Reference
Love, Medicine and Miracles by Bernie Siegel. Ebury House (1999).

E is for Exercise

Scientists believe that taking regular exercise can reduce the risk of developing cancer dramatically. Researchers at the University of Bristol suggest that physical activity can cut the risk of bowel cancer and may help prevent breast, prostate, lung and endometrial cancer. Moreover, for cancer patients, regular exercise can improve their feeling of well-being and overall strength, increasing their ability to withstand the treatments required and to remain positive in the fight against the disease.

For a patient recovering from an operation or the effects of chemotherapy, Eastern exercise practices may be particularly appropriate (see 'Q is for Qigong'; 'T is for Tai Chi'; 'Y is for Yoga'), integrated holistic practices that stimulate the body and rebalance the system. Ideally some form of aerobic exercise should be taken, say 30 minutes twice a week. But where this is not realistic at the early stage of the recovery process, a stretching routine may be more appropriate.

It is a misconception that exercise should be avoided during radiotherapy or chemotherapy. Light and stimulating exercise, even if very gentle, helps reduce fatigue caused by treatment, increases the sense of self-empowerment, improves psychological well-being, and lowers anxiety and the risk of depression. Exercise and the advantages it brings can promote a more positive outlook and help make cancer just a part of your life, not all of it.

TOP TIPS

By remaining as fit as possible, by continuing to pursue hobbies and by participating in classes such as aerobics or yoga, you can regain some control and feel so much better for it.

Listen to your body and consult your medical teams to find the best exercise regime to complement your treatment.

Further information

UK

NACER (National Association of Cancer Exercise Rehabilitation) Tel: 01789 555675. Website: www.nacer.org.uk

Anti-cancer: A New Way of Life by David Servan-Schreiber. Michael Joseph (2008). Available from **Penny Brohn Cancer Care**: www.shopatpennybrohn.com/product1796.asp?PageID=53

US

National Cancer Institute: Guidelines Urge Exercise for Cancer Patients, Survivors: www.cancer.gov/ncicancerbulletin/062910/page5

Exercise programmes for cancer patients are popping up all over the country. This page from the **American Cancer Society** lists a few examples: www.cancer.org/docroot/MIT/content/MIT_2_4X_Exercise_Programs_Benefit_Cancer_Patients_Recovery.asp

Gilda's Club and the **Wellness Community** often offer free exercise programmes for cancer patients, as well as activities and support groups: For Gilda's Clubs, see: www.gildasclub.org/findaclubhouse.asp. For Wellness Community programmes, see: www.thewellnesscommunity.org/corporate/facilities.php

F is for Faith

Faith is living your life as though God is there all the time, on a continuous and daily basis. Any good relationship is nurtured by trust and the same is true with God. It is rather like a husband or wife who have lived lovingly together for many years. They live their life in the consciousness of the other's presence. Often it will all seem routine and straightforward. But there will also be times when the stakes are high and full of pressure.

The normal rhythm of faith means going about your day wanting to please the Lord in whom you trust. It makes a difference to how you behave and to how you react to things good and bad. It will temper your responses and your attitude to your daily tasks. The poet, George Herbert, put it in a nutshell:

Teach me, my God and King,

In all things Thee to see;

And what I do in anything

To do it as for Thee.

He sees faith as a kind of alchemy which lights up the routine and fills everyday life with glory.

This is the famous stone

That turneth all to gold

For that which God doth touch and own

Cannot for less be told.

It has been well said that it is how we act in the little things that often leaves the biggest impression. But there are also times in the life of faith when we need to go out on a limb for God. Perhaps we face a crisis of which we cannot see the outcome or the way through. We feel exposed and vulnerable. Yet we know that God is still there with us and has never let us down. Our faith tells us that He loves us so much that Christ died for us, and that, having given so much for us, He won't fail us now. We have an inner confidence, an assurance that He has prepared a way and that He will see us through. At such times of vulnerability we can know the truest peace.

Further information
UK
CANCERactive, 'Prayer and Cancer Healing: The Power of Prayer to Heal': www.canceractive.com/cancer-active-page-link.aspx?n=458

US
National Cancer Institute information on spirituality and cancer: www.cancer.gov/cancertopics/pdq/supportivecare/spirituality/Patient

American Cancer Society, information on spirituality and prayer: www.cancer.org/Treatment/TreatmentsandSideEffects/Complementary andAlternativeMedicine/MindBodyandSpirit/spirituality-and-prayer

References
Anatomy of the Spirit: The Seven Stages of Power and Healing by Caroline Myss. Bantam (1997).

Reflections on Spirituality and Health by Stephen Wright. Wiley-Blackwell (2005).

F is for Fatigue

There are four main causes of fatigue: the disease, the treatment, the emotional rollercoaster and the fact that you are just plain tired. Forget having children to feed and a report to prepare. This is the moment to put your own welfare first. If you are tired – rest.

Sometimes fatigue is an indicator that all is not well and that disease is present. Cancer stresses your body's normal way of functioning: rapid production of cancer cells uses more energy, leaving you tired and depleted. If there is pain, it is even more exhausting. And worrying about the disease may be causing sleepless nights. Treatment – whether it be surgery, chemotherapy, radiation or all of the above – is also likely to cause tiredness. An intravenous injection of vitamin C can be very helpful, together with homeopathy and naturopathy. But you must ensure that the doctors treating you know absolutely everything you are taking.

There is usually a pattern to the fatigue associated with chemotherapy, whether it occurs on the first day or two after the treatment, or a week to ten days later when the white blood cell count might be at its lowest.

I experienced extreme fatigue while taking chemotherapy, so much so that I usually slept through the entire treatment. I usually fell asleep as the Piriton (an antihistamine given before chemo to prevent an allergic reaction to paclitaxel) was being injected. Such medications are sedating and this sedation can last – a bit like a hangover.

I do not remember experiencing fatigue during radiotherapy. But since cancer cells are being killed off, and the kidneys and liver are working harder to eliminate the toxins from the body, it would be surprising not to feel tired. I remember I did drink much more water than usual during this time.

Although you may feel too tired to exercise, that may be exactly what you need to do. Lethargy, easily confused with fatigue, can set in if you have not managed at least a little gentle exercise and fresh air. If fatigue becomes all-consuming, then it is time to alert the professionals – help is at hand.

TOP TIPS

Get a good night's sleep by fair means (hot chocolate before bedtime) or foul (Nytol, the over-the-counter sleeping tablet, or something stronger from the doctor if the problem persists). Do not tolerate sleepless nights since your fatigue will become worse. Remember that your body is best able to get on with healing itself when you are most relaxed and asleep. Allocate yourself a full twelve hours for a good night's sleep.

The logistics of making extra time in the day for medical appointments adds to fatigue. Getting there, parking the car, long waits because the appointment system has gone awry – all take their toll. So let a friend do the driving. If there are any delays to your treatment, then do some shopping or read a book. Use the time profitably – monitor, manage, and remember there are some things you *can* control.

Further information

UK

Macmillan Cancer Support: www.macmillan.org.uk/Cancerinformation/
Livingwithandaftercancer/Symptomssideeffects/Fatigue/Effects.aspx

US

An excellent list of online resources from **Fighting Cancer Fatigue** about
cancer fatigue (includes sites from both UK and US): www.cancerfatigue.
org/resources-cancer-fatigue.php

The **University of Maryland Medical Center** provides tips for good sleep
hygiene: www.umm.edu/sleep/sleep_hyg.htm

F is for Fear

Facing the diagnosis of cancer is facing neat, unadulterated fear.
Fear of the unknown – what is going to happen? am I going to
suffer? Fear of death – am I going to die and when? And fear of
change – life will never again be the same. The irrational mind
overtakes the rational.

But fear lives in uncertainty. When you *know* what is going
to happen – that you will be treated as an outpatient or in
hospital; that you will be advised and counselled; that you will
have maybe an operation, or chemotherapy, or radiotherapy – it
all becomes doable. Family and friends flock round to support
you. Associates turn from being impossible to being kind. You
meet some fantastically dedicated people working in our health
service. And then you look back and wonder what there was to
fear.

When fear of dying and suffering is unpacked, the reality
is that sophisticated drugs mean no one needs to die in pain.
Suffering – another fearsome word, but definitely unpackable
– is a matter of degree. Fear of not seeing a family grow up or
leaving a loved one is not really fear but deep disappointment.
And there is very good reason not to let fear get a grip because
of the immune system suppression it may cause.

To some, the fear of change is far greater than others. My sisters and I absolutely hate and fear change. Paula has the most fantastic boyfriend – but will she move in with him? Only if she can overcome this fear. Sara's husband died, and one day she was too frightened to leave the house. It sounds completely ludicrous. But I have been exactly where Paula is, and when I was divorced from my first husband, I felt exactly the same way as Sara. I used to sit and cry because I was so frightened of the change and what life might hold.

The diagnosis of cancer allowed me to embrace change. And this is the key. Is your life so great on all fronts that you would not like to see some changes? Here is your big chance. One little change of a 'g' to a 'c' and you have chances, not changes. In my view, that deals with that particular fear.

From a doctor's viewpoint, it adds to difficulties if the patient is consumed with fear – because he's got the 'bogey-man' to deal with as well as the disease. The doctor can either fuel the fear by emphasizing the poor prognosis or, while not promising cure, stress all those actions he is going to recommend to stop the tumour in its tracks.

TOP TIP

Fear is like a balloon – keep blowing and it gets bigger; take a pin and burst it, and there's nothing inside.

Further information
UK

Cancer Research UK has helpful information on fear, anxiety and panic and lists of counselling organizations to contact for advice and support: www.cancerhelp.org.uk/coping-with-cancer/coping-emotionally/cancer-and-your-emotions

US

The **American Cancer Society** has excellent information on anxiety and fear: www.cancer.org/Treatment/TreatmentsandSideEffects/PhysicalSideEffects/DealingwithSymptomsatHome/caring-for-the-patient-with-cancer-at-home-anxiety-and-fear; 'Living with Uncertainty: The Fear of Cancer Recurrence': www.cancer.org/Treatment/SurvivorshipDuringandAfterTreatment/UnderstandingRecurrence/LivingWithUncertainty/living-with-uncertainty-toc

F is for Flower Essences

A
B
C
D
E
F
G
H
I
J
K
L
M
N
O
P
Q
R
S
T
U
V
W
X
Y
Z

The most famous flower essences are those of Dr Edward Bach. He believed that personality traits and moods had a direct effect on the body and were the underlying cause of disease. This belief led him to the study of immunology and his subsequent appointment as pathologist and bacteriologist at the London Homeopathic Hospital.

Devoting himself during the 1930s to researching flower remedies, he observed early morning sunlight passing through dewdrops on flower petals and concluded that water might retain the energy and healing power of the flower. This led to his practice of picking flowers and floating them in spring water in full sunshine for a few hours to obtain the 'mother tincture' from which, once diluted and preserved in alcohol, the bottled essence was made. In the absence of sunlight, he would boil the petals in water and preserve the essence in brandy.

Bach believed that the 'energetic' nature of the flower could be transmitted to the user to overcome negative feelings and restore balance and harmony. When experiencing a negative emotion, Bach was reported to have suspended his hand above various plants. If he felt relief from the emotion whilst doing so over a particular plant, he would attribute the power to heal the specific emotional problem to that plant. Over six years he intuitively developed a complete system of 38 essences for treating easily recognizable emotional and spiritual conditions including insomnia, stress, anxiety, depression, fear and anger, and their underlying causes.

The best-known Bach flower remedy is 'Rescue Remedy' – an emergency combination containing five flower remedies: Impatiens, Cherry Plum, Rock Rose, Star of Bethlehem and Clematis. Recommended for times of crisis, it is believed to be excellent for reducing fear, nervousness and tension. 'Rescue Cream' is also available for external use.

More recently, Dr Arthur Bailey, a scientist and chartered engineer, discovered dowsing and flower essence healing when taking early retirement due to ME. He systematically used dowsing to produce a set of flower essences concentrating on issues of self-esteem, personal development and liberation from negative belief systems. The main emphasis of his flower essences is to act as catalysts for change, treating attitudes of mind and negative thought patterns rather than acting on the emotional plane. His wide range of essences for helping to integrate mind, body and spirit include the roadside Blue Pimpernel, for 're-awakening our links with the source of our being', Red Clover for releasing emotional blockages and the Himalayan Blue Poppy for discovering your life's purpose and fulfilling your potential.

TOP TIP

If you send a small hair sample to them, Bailey Flower Essences will dowse to decide which flower essences would be most appropriate for you. Alternatively, if you feel like trying this out for yourself, a short course in using a pendulum to dowse is available on their website www.baileyessences.com.

Further information
UK

Bailey Flower Essences, 7 Nelson Road, Ilkley, West Yorkshire LS29 8HN Tel: 01943 432012. Website: www.baileyessences.com

Bach Flower Therapy, The Bach Centre, Mount Vernon, Bakers Lane, Brightwell-cum-Sotwell, Oxfordshire OX10 0PZ. Tel: 01491 834678. Website: www.bachcentre.com

References
Anyone Can Dowse for Better Health by Arthur Bailey. W. Foulsham & Co (1998).

The Handbook of Bailey Flower Essences by Arthur Bailey. Blue Ocean Publishing (2009).

Illustrated Handbook of the Bach Flower Remedies by Phillip M. Chancellor. Vermilion (2005).

F is for Folic Acid

Folic acid, also known as folate or folacin, is an essential B vitamin that helps prevent birth defects and promotes good health.

Folic acid was given this name by the nutritionist Roger Williams because of its presence in the dark green foliage of vegetables such as kale and spinach. Folate refers specifically to the form of folic acid found naturally in food, as opposed to forms of folic acid found in supplements. Folate occurs in meats such as beef, lamb and pork, and in wholewheat, asparagus and broccoli. Even when present in foods, much is lost in cooking, and natural folates lose their effectiveness relatively rapidly over a period of days or weeks as they are chemically unstable. (Synthetic folic acid in contrast is stable for a far longer period.) Also, the body may have difficulty in absorbing folate. Folic acid in supplements or when added to foods may be more easily absorbed. The amount of folate stored in the body is best reflected in the folate concentration in red blood cells.

Folic acid, although best known for its use in preventing the serious birth defect spina bifida, participates in a huge variety of biochemical reactions including the production of red and white blood cells and DNA. It also has a significant role in supporting the immune system. Many consider that folic acid could be used in moderate doses to help in the battle to fight cancer, particularly of the colon and cervix. As opinions are divided on this subject, the use of folic acid should be discussed with your medical team.

TOP TIP

Folate is found naturally in many foods included in a healthy diet. In addition to those mentioned above, folic acid is found in breakfast cereals, lentils, tomato juice, brussels sprouts and oranges. (See 'D is for Diet and Nutritional Therapy (or Food, Glorious Food)'.)

Further information

US

In the herbs and supplements section of **Lewis Gale Hospital** website there is excellent information on folic acid. Scroll down to 'Natural and Alternative Treatments' on the main menu and click on 'Herbs and Supplements'. Then find 'Folic acid' in the A–Z list: www.alleghanyregional.com/healthcontent. asp?page=contentselection/condensedmainindex

Information from **Memorial Sloan-Kettering Cancer Center** on folic acid: www.mskcc.org/mskcc/html/69225.cfm

Reference

Folic Acid: Essential for Prenatal Health by Allan Spreen. Woodland Publishing (2000).

F is for Food

See 'D is for Diet and Nutritional Therapy (or Food, Glorious Food)'

F is for Friend

To be the friend of someone diagnosed or living with cancer is not a particularly easy role. But if you are determined to stand by them, here are a few tips.

First, help with the logistics of life. When a person is not feeling that energized, to drive to the hospital, park, get to the appointment and drive home again can take a huge effort. So volunteering to be the driver for a day is a very good present. So too is collecting the children from school, giving them tea and overseeing homework. Given the importance of diet, help with the shopping or popping in at lunch time *with a lunch* or something for dinner that only needs reheating is all so helpful.

Even the simplest chores can feel like climbing humungous mountains. Help clearing up the breakfast, making the beds or collecting prescriptions can mean that needed rest and relaxation will be the order of the day. Continuing to work is not necessarily bad, but anything that can be done to alleviate peripheral stress – such as a lift to and from work – is helpful. And a friend in the workplace is a friend indeed.

Often the burden of cancer can be huge. You feel almost as if a smile would crack your face and that your very personality is being subsumed by this great weight of glumness. So the best friend is one who by sheer effort of will and personality can make the sun shine through the dark clouds. A funny conversation on the telephone can be hugely uplifting. The suggestion of an afternoon of cinema or ice-skating or tennis can lift the mood completely.

But beware crossing the fine line between sympathy and being patronizing, between the humorous and the flippant, between an approach that is positive and one that is uncompassionate. People with cancer are vulnerable, no matter how strong and brave they may appear. They are sensitive, so tread gently. If you are known for your big feet, imagine them in tiny shoes treading gently through a meadow and not squashing the poppies!

TOP TIP

Be the friend you would want and need if the shoes were on the other foot!

Further information

UK

CANCERactive Tel: 01280 821211. Visit the website for their support group directory: www.canceractive.com

The **BBC Health** site gives practical advice for supporting a friend or relative with cancer: www.bbc.co.uk/health/support/supportcancer_family.shtml

US

To organize friend support teams online see **Lotsa Helping Hands**: www. lotsahelpinghands.com, and **CaringBridge**: www.caringbridge.org

Ideas for supporting a friend who has cancer from the **American Society of Oncology**: http://origin.cancer.net/patient/All+About+Cancer/Cancer. Net+Feature+Articles/Family,+Friends,+and+Caregivers/Supporting+a+ Friend+Who+Has+Cancer

Reference

What Can I do to Help? 75 Practical Ideas for Family and Friends from Cancer's Frontline by Deborah Hutton. Short Books (2005).

G is for Garlic

Garlic has long been used as a healing herb. Allicin (thought by many to be the most important active ingredient in garlic) is known for its antibiotic, healing, cleansing and immune-boosting properties and so is often recommended for people affected by cancer. Recent research has suggested that garlic can trigger apoptosis (cancer cell death). It is thought that garlic might interfere with cancer cell multiplication and metastasis. It is held to be an anti-inflammatory, to have antioxidant properties, and to protect the liver and support enzymes which eliminate carcinogenic toxins from the body. This all seems like very good news. But, to be effective, it appears that the garlic must be fresh, crushed and eaten raw.

TOP TIP

There is little more delicious than dunking wholemeal brown bread into olive oil (cold pressed) in which garlic has been crushed and soaked. Fresh parsley needs to be on standby and chewed to freshen the breath.

Further information

UK

See the *Daily Mail's* article, 'Is garlic a "cure-all"?': www.dailymail.co.uk/health/article-4954/Is-garlic-cure-all.html

CANCERactive: www.canceractive.com/cancer-active-page-link.aspx?n=525&Title=Garlic

US

Information on garlic including contraindications and drug interaction is available from the **Lewis Gale Hospital** website. Scroll down to 'Natural and Alternative Treatments' on the main menu and click on 'Herbs and Supplements'. Then find 'Garlic' in the A–Z list: www.alleghanyregional.com/health content.asp?page=contentselection/condensedmainindex

Memorial Sloan-Kettering Cancer Center: www.mskcc.org/mskcc/html/69230.cfm

ConsumerLab in the US tests garlic supplements for content and contaminants: www.consumerlab.com

Reference

The Heart of Garlic: Allicin's Effective Natural Healing Properties by Peter Josling. Natural Health Holdings (2003).

G is for Genes and Gene Therapy

At a crucial stage in evolution, single-celled organisms turned into multicellular forms of life. For the first time, an individual cell had to be aware of what other cells were doing. It had to know when it should divide and when it should not. Whole new chapters had to be written into the DNA code book as certain genes developed with the job of controlling the activity of others: in simple terms, they were on/off switches. If these switches developed faults, or if they became separated from the genes they were supposed to manage, uncontrolled growth – cancer – could result.

Twenty years ago, that was an important insight, and one of its results was an enthusiasm for gene therapy. The idea was that if we could replace the faulty growth-suppressing gene in a cancer cell, we could cure the disease. The theory was good, and there was a great deal of interest in replacing a specific gene called p53 which is often mutated and so ineffective in cancer cells. But, in practice, attempts to replace such defective growth-control genes have been disappointing. So too has the idea that we might be able to use viruses to carry a 'suicide gene' into cancer cells that would selectively activate a toxic drug. There may be greater promise in efforts to introduce genes into cancer cells that will provoke our immune system into killing them. But most of the work has not moved beyond the stage of using laboratory animals or cancer cells in a dish. As for the treatment of cancer patients with any form of gene therapy, this is still possible only in the setting of a clinical trial.

Researchers have faced many difficulties. It is not easy to find viruses that will infect only cancer cells, and it is difficult to predict the place in the cell's genetic material where the virus will insert its genes (including the one that it has been engineered to smuggle in). Understandable concern that genetically modified organisms might escape from a lab or hospital and infect the wider population means that gene therapy studies can be conducted only under the most carefully controlled conditions.

Gene therapy for cancer may be some way off. But our knowledge about the genetic basis of the disease is already paying dividends. Identifying the precise genetic mutations that have occurred in a particular tumour is beginning to guide treatment in lung cancer, for example. In this disease, faulty control of a specific kind of growth receptor on the cell surface predicts tumour shrinkage when the drugs erlotinib and gefitinib are given (see 'D is for Drugs (Targeted Drugs)').

Such developments bring the prospect of tailoring treatment to the characteristics of the cancer in each individual patient. Personalized therapy will also eventually involve assessing someone's likely susceptibiity to different side effects. This will again involve knowing their genetic make-up. And of course we are already using our knowledge about cancer-causing genes to help people understand their risk of developing a particular kind of tumour, such as the inherited form of breast cancer (see 'B is for BRCA1 and BRCA2'). So genes will guide prevention as well as treatment.

Further information

UK

Search for 'gene therapy' at **Cancer Research UK**: www.cancerresearchuk. org

US

National Cancer Institute, 'Gene Therapy for Cancer: Questions and Answers': www.cancer.gov/cancertopics/factsheet/Therapy/gene

G is for Gerson Therapy

Max Gerson (1881–1959) developed the Gerson method of naturopathic cancer treatment. Dr Gerson first attracted the friendship of Nobel Prize Laureate Albert Schweitzer by curing his wife of tuberculosis after all conventional treatments had failed. Later, Schweitzer's own type 2 diabetes was cured by Gerson's therapy. Schweitzer said of his friend, 'I see in Dr Gerson one of the most eminent geniuses in the history of medicine.'

Gerson Therapy takes a holistic view of so-called 'incurable' conditions including cancer, diabetes, arthritis and other degenerative diseases. The primary objective of this nutritional therapy is *to activate the body's ability to heal itself* through cellular regeneration, particularly of the liver, and a restored immune system.

The therapy is intended to work in the following way. First, it boosts the immune system and helps the body break down diseased tissue by bombarding it with enzymes, nutrients and minerals from 13 glasses of organically sourced, double-pressed raw juice per day. Second, once the immune system is functioning, the treatment eliminates the toxins from broken-down tumours and diseased tissues through a regime of daily coffee enemas. The caffeine in the enemas is absorbed by the liver, stimulating it to excrete the filtered toxins naturally by increased flow of bile through the opened liver/bile ducts.

Advocating a low-fat, low-protein diet similar to that of our cave-dwelling ancestors – together with various supplements, vitamins and digestive enzymes – the therapy also addresses the sodium/potassium imbalances that occur in cancer sufferers. Potassium is boosted and sodium eliminated.

Max Gerson said, 'Stay close to nature and its eternal laws will protect you.' He considered that degenerative diseases are caused by toxic, degraded food, water and air. The therapy strongly recommends drinking purified water, consuming organically grown food, and avoiding contact with pollutants by using only natural household and personal toiletries to reduce toxin build-up in the body.

Charlotte Gerson continues her father's work. In 1977, she founded the Gerson Institute in San Diego, licensing the methodology to hospitals and clinics, referring patients to licensed treatment centres in Mexico and Hungary, and training health professionals, patients and others who wish to learn the regime. Since the treatment is complex and requires significant attention to detail to achieve the best results, the Institute recommends that patients should start their therapy at a centre licensed by the Institute.

The organization makes very clear that following the rigorous regime of hourly juicing, enemas and diet requires a high level of physical, practical and financial commitment from both the patient and the carer. There is further information on the websites below. Before embarking on the therapy, it may be helpful to read *A Time to Heal* by Beata Bishop. This is the compelling story of how she beat malignant melanoma 23 years ago by following the strict dietary regime.

According to the Gerson Support Group UK, patients undergoing chemotherapy may choose to adopt and benefit from some elements of the Gerson Diet, and recommend a maximum of three glasses of freshly made juice and one coffee enema a day. They stress that this is *not* the same as following Gerson Therapy. The two approaches are considered strongly contradictory: chemotherapy uses toxic drugs, and Gerson Therapy aims to detoxify the body.

Where chemotherapy has been unsuccessful, the Gerson Institute strongly encourages patients to visit a Gerson treatment centre and *not* begin the therapy at home. It is essential that the liver is not placed under too great stress by the overly quick release of toxins and chemotherapy residues into the blood. Doctors can slow the process down by regulating the amount of juice consumed and the frequency of enemas. A protocol tailored to each patient's needs provides advice on how the therapy can be continued at home, along with contact information for caregivers and support.

I made the decision to embark on a course of chemotherapy but was impressed by Charlotte Gerson's remarkable conviction when speaking at a conference in London. Whilst deciding not to follow the regime, I was aware of growing evidence that fruit and vegetables do indeed have an immune-boosting effect, and help to maintain levels of important nutrients and improve digestive transit, which can be impaired as a side effect of chemotherapy. I complemented my already largely organic diet with a daily breakfast juice of organic carrot, broccoli and apple with a little ginger to soothe any nausea – again a side effect of the chemotherapy (see 'J is for Juicing').

Leading cancer specialists are cautious and often sceptical in their attitude to Gerson Therapy. Many more studies and much more evidence are required before it can be accepted that diet, including high doses of vitamin C and enemas, can destroy tumours. They do, however, recognize growing evidence of the role of nutrition in general in preventing and treating cancer.

Further information
UK

The **Gerson Support Group**, PO Box 406, Esher, Surrey KT10 9UL. Helpline: 01372 464557. Website: www.gersonsupportgroup.org.uk

CANCERactive: www.canceractive.com

UK Juicers: www.ukjuicers.com/comparingjuicers.htm

US

The **Gerson Institute's** website includes studies and case histories: www.gerson.org

National Cancer Institute information on Gerson Therapy: www.cancer.gov/cancertopics/pdq/cam/gerson/Patient/page2

For a thorough review of the Gerson Treatment, see **Quackwatch**: www.quackwatch.org/01QuackeryRelatedTopics/OTA/ota03.html

Norwalk Juicers: www.norwalkjuicers.com

References

The Little Green Juicing Book by the Gerson Support Group (to order see contact details above).

The Gerson Therapy: The Proven Nutritional Program for Cancer and Other Illnesses by Charlotte Gerson and Morton Walker. Kensington (2005).

A Cancer Therapy: Results of Fifty Cases and the Cure of Advanced Cancer by Diet Therapy by Max Gerson. The Gerson Institute (originally published 1958, now in its 6th Edition).

Healing the Gerson Way: Defeating Cancer and Other Chronic Diseases by Charlotte Gerson and Beata Bishop. Totality Books (2007).

A Time to Heal: Triumph over Cancer – The Therapy of the Future by Beata Bishop. Penguin (1999).

A
B
C
D
E
F
G
H
I
J
K
L
M
N
O
P
Q
R
S
T
U
V
W
X
Y
Z

A
B
C
D
E
F
G
H
I
J
K
L
M
N
O
P
Q
R
S
T
U
V
W
X
Y
Z

H is for Hair Loss

Some people deal with this much better than others. For men, it's quite sexy. For some women it is a means to an end: the chemo or radiotherapy that causes hair loss is potentially life-saving, and therefore hair loss is a small price to pay. This tends to be the approach of the medical profession. But it can be particularly irritating when expressed by some smug, pompous, inexperienced junior registrar, who, in the context of cancer, thinks loss of hair is a mere incidental. And, after all, it does not actually affect your health. Wrong, wrong, wrong.

This is wrong, in the first instance, because not all chemotherapy causes loss of hair. You need to ask whether this will happen before agreeing to the proposed drug. With the new range of targeted therapies, it may be possible to choose a drug which does not cause hair loss.

Wrong – because you can quite easily live with a diagnosis of cancer, but with hair loss you are a marked woman (see 'W is for Wigs'). Men, of course, often go bald and are not marked out as having cancer.

Wrong – because what you look like *does* affect how you feel, and how you feel affects your health. Any junior registrar who has not engaged with that simplest of facts should give up all ideas of being a doctor. And watch out for the nasty little junior registrar who tries to frighten you by saying 'Your hair will probably grow back after chemo', thereby putting into your mind a little doubt that you will ever see it again! After chemo, hair always grows back. (It is only after radiotherapy to the brain that there can be a problem.)

Having suffered the hair loss, there is the matter of the hair growing back. In my case, there was damage to the hair follicle, and it grew back in tight greyish curls. Gradually, over a period of six months, it grew as normal – dead straight. And when I eventually braved my hairdresser, he confirmed it was in beautiful condition, really healthy and strong. This may have been because I had put into practice this very serious regime:

1. *No chemicals; no perming/dyeing.*

2. *No brushing (have a short haircut which can be styled by running fingers through it).*

3. *No pulling of any kind – avoid hairbrush, rollers, tongs, even strong winds (wear a hat).*

4. *No heat – no hairdryers, tongs, electric rollers, blow drys.*

5. *No unnecessary washing of the hair – essential only; shake and pat dry.*

6. *Keep scalp well moisturized with natural oils and hair conditioned only with natural products.*

7. *If you absolutely have to dye your hair, use only natural dyes and loads of conditioner.*

8. *Take a herbal supplement for your hair and nails.*

9. *Try not to lose your hair in the first place – the cold cap is not 100% guaranteed to work but does for some (see 'C is for Cold Cap').*

10. *If you do lose your hair and look good in hats, there is a great range of both winter warm hats and summer straw! And see 'W is for Wigs'.*

TOP TIPS

For all those junior registrars, the right approach to hair loss is absolute and utter sympathy and support (rather than sneering and snotty remarks!), together with resounding comfort and maximum charm. Do not be under any illusion – for some, hair loss is a truly miserable experience.

Further information
UK

For information on obtaining a wig through the National Health Service or privately, and a list of companies that supply wigs, hats and scarves, see **Cancer Research UK**: www.cancerhelp.org.uk/about-cancer/cancer-questions/hair-loss-and-wigs

US

For a list of US retailers supplying wigs and hair loss accessories directly, see **American Cancer Society**: www.cancer.org/Cancer/BreastCancer/MoreInformation/breast-prostheses-and-hair-loss-accessories-list

Some US insurance companies provide reimbursement for wigs if you have a prescription for one from your oncologist. Check your insurance benefits.

H is for Healing

See 'M is for Mind, Body, Spirit and Healing'

H is for Herbal (Phytotherapeutic) Medicine

Herbal medicines or remedies can be made from a plant's leaves, flowers, seeds or roots, alone or in combination. Strictly speaking, a herb is not a tree, yet many well-known herbal medicines derive from trees. Not least is slippery elm powder, which comes from the bark of the slippery elm tree (*Ulmus rubra*). (See also 'A is for Aloe Vera'; 'A is for Astragalus'; 'C is for Cat's Claw'; 'C is for Carctol'; 'E is for Echinacea'; 'E is for Essiac'; 'G is for Garlic'; 'M is for Mistletoe'.)

In many cases, drugs used in orthodox medicine arise in one way or another from plants. The most obvious example is morphine, which is made from the opium poppy. Another example is the heart drug digitalis, found in foxgloves. But many examples are less well known. Sometimes pharmaceutical companies continue to extract the active ingredients from plants and herbs. In other cases, they work out the substance's chemical structure and then synthesize it in the laboratory. There are examples among chemotherapy drugs. The 'taxane' class of drugs, used to treat breast and lung cancers, for example, is so called because the botanical name for the yew tree is 'taxus'. Paclitaxel (Taxol) was extracted originally from the leaves of the Pacific yew (*Taxus brevifolia*) and docetaxel (Taxotere) was first isolated from the common European yew (*Taxus baccata*). Both drugs are now synthesized.

There are many herbs that can help cancer patients, and my own experience provides a good illustration. I was taking part in a clinical trial of the breast cancer drug lapatinib (Tykerb) and I was struggling with a particularly vicious attack of cramps, diarrhoea and a deeply unpleasant burning sensation. It was suggested that I took a teaspoon of slippery elm powder on my muesli in the morning. The problems stopped completely, and I was able to tolerate the drug well.

Many herbs contain powerful antioxidants, which makes them useful as part of a regime aimed at keeping well during cancer treatment. Although we should note that some evidence suggests the use of antioxidants during cancer treatment is unwise since – at least in theory – they may help the survival of cancerous (as well as healthy) cells (see the article by Brian Lawrence and colleagues in 'References' on the following page). Other herbs aid the body's pathways of elimination: examples include laxatives, diuretics, expectorants for the respiratory system, and those offering support to the liver and lymphatic system.

The herbal approach can also help with emotional and hormonal problems as well as depression, mood swings, poor memory and insomnia – all of which can be an issue before, during or after cancer treatment. Once treatment has been completed, consulting a herbalist may offer a way of optimizing health and energy, helping you on your path to well-being.

TOP TIP

Some books encourage herbal treatment by self-prescription. This can only be described as very dangerous for a cancer patient since herbal remedies can interact badly with conventional medicines. It is essential for your oncologist or other doctor to liaise with your herbalist. As long as your herbalist is properly qualified, there should be no problem with this.

Further information
UK

British Herbal Medicine Association, PO Box 583, Exeter EX1 9GX. Tel: 01202 433691. Email: secretary@bhma.info. Website: www.bhma.info

Register of Chinese Herbal Medicine, 1 Exeter Street, Norwich NR2. 4QB Tel: 01603 623994. Website: www.rchm.co.uk

National Institute of Medical Herbalists, Elm House, 54 Mary Arches Street, Exeter EX4 3BA. Tel: 01392 426022. Website: www.nimh.org.uk

US

Not all herbal medicines and supplements contain the listed ingredients in the amounts described, and some may be contaminated. Several organizations provide reliable information derived from independent testing. There is a cost for subscribing to these services but the cost is worthwhile if you are seriously exploring herbal supplements. See **ConsumerLab** at www.consumerlab.com and **Consumer Reports** Natural Health Guide at www.consumerreports.org/health/natural-health.htm

For general informaton on herbs and supplements, including research findings, contraindications and drug interactions, see **Lewis Gale Hospital** website: www.alleghanyregional.com/healthcontent.asp?page=contentselection/condensedmainindex. Scroll down to 'Natural and Alternative Treatments' on the main menu, click on 'NAT index', then browse through the 'Herbs and Supplements' section.

References

Herbs Against Cancer: History and Controversy by Ralph W. Moss. Equinox Press (1998).

Encylopedia of Herbal Medicine by Thomas Bartram. Grace (1995).

Holistic Herbal: A Safe and Practical Guide to Making and Using Herbal Remedies by David Hoffman. Thorsons (2002).

'Should supplemental antioxidant administration be avoided during chemotherapy and radiation therapy?' by Brian Lawrence and colleagues, *Journal of the National Cancer Institute 2008*, volume 100, pages 773–783: http://bit.ly/9nQnts.

H is for Histology

Typically, doctors remove a small part of the suspicious tissue (see 'B is for Biopsy'), or sometimes the whole tumour, and then have it cut into thin sections and examined under a microscope in the laboratory. This examination is termed histology. It is usual for the tissue to be stained so that the way the cells are arranged can easily be seen. The histologist looks to see whether growth has been orderly, as in normal tissue, or anarchic and invasive, as in cancer.

The overall appearance of the tissue is usually sufficient to answer the fundamental question about whether the growth is benign or malignant – but there are different degrees of malignancy. Some cancers are made up of cells that – despite abnormal features – still resemble healthy cells from the same tissue. Such cells are said to be well differentiated (or low-grade). These cells grow relatively slowly and are less likely to spread to other parts of the body. Poorly differentiated cells, on the other hand, have lost almost all the characteristics of healthy cells. Tumours formed of these cells tend to grow rapidly and spread quickly, and are termed high-grade.

The detailed way in which histologists grade and describe tumours varies from one cancer to another. In the case of prostate cancer, for example, cancers are given what is called the 'Gleason score'. But the principle is the same: high-grade tumours are likely to be more aggressive than low-grade ones. Along with other factors, such as the size of the original tumour and the extent to which it has already spread – if it has spread at all – tumour grade helps doctors suggest a plan for treatment that best suits the individual patient.

Where there is concern that the cancer may have spread, it is usual to remove lymph nodes that could be affected. These too will be examined by the histologist to see if tumour cells are present.

For some cancers, histology can provide other valuable information. In the case of breast cancer, histologists stain tumour cells to see if they have on their surface receptors for the hormones oestrogen and progesterone. This has important implications for treatment (see 'H is for Hormone Therapy').

Histologists are now also asked to establish whether a patient's breast cancer cells have too many of a kind of receptor called HER2. If such receptors are overexpressed on a cell, it keeps receiving the signal to divide. Tumours which are positive for HER2 are likely to respond to the drug trastuzumab (Herceptin), which blocks the faulty receptor. There is a range of other factors controlling cell growth, and our knowledge of how they stimulate many different kinds of cancer – and how blocking them can provide effective treatment – is a fast-growing area of medicine.

H is for Holistic

This is a much used but not always well-understood term. It does not signify holiness in the religious sense, although it does not exclude this, since holism is a mind–body–spirit approach. Sometimes it is misspelt as 'wholistic', and this spelling is perhaps more true to its meaning, which encompasses the 'whole body' – not just the physical but the spiritual and mental also. In *The Healer's Manual*, Ted Andrews writes, 'Health is the ideal balance between all major parts of our being – body, mind and soul – in conjunction with our environment and all we encounter' (see page 3 of book in 'References' on the following page).

So a holistic diet is a diet which nourishes the mind, the body and the spirit or soul. Holistic medicine is medicine which is practised having care for, or treating, the whole body, mind and spirit of the patient.

This is not necessarily in line with medicine as generally practised. If you go to the doctor, you usually have a specific complaint – say a twisted ankle – in which case you would not expect to have a conversation about your spiritual health: you would expect an X-ray and some painkillers. But the very nature of cancer demands a holistic approach. Cancer which appears in the breast can spread to the lymph nodes, or to the lungs; the very blood which courses through lung and breast is also coursing through the liver, and with it the signals of disease. *My whole body, my mind and my spirit know I have cancer and so for me there is no debate: cancer treatment has to be holistic.*

Medical training in this country emphasizes proof of safety and efficacy. To obtain scientific evidence, the body has been 'methodologically unpacked': each part has been singled out, dissected, studied, tested. Specialisms have developed. The basis of our approach is the individual problem, the individual broken part; and we have not generally been overly concerned about that part – until it breaks or fails us. If we look at all at the relationship of the broken part to the whole, it is only when the part has gone wrong.

But cancer *is* a whole-body disease. This is one of the reasons it is such a challenge to the medical profession, and why it really is a life-changing experience, not just for the patient but for all those involved in cancer care. Cancer calls into question the very essence of the medical approach. That said, the past few years have seen huge shifts in thinking, not least in the integration of complementary therapies alongside orthodox medical care. Another fascinating aspect is that we do, of course, have the technical and scientific means to test the efficacy of some of the ancient holistic healing practices. Acupuncture is a compelling example.

TOP TIP
Holistic medicine does not exclude orthodox medicine.

Further information
References

Testing Treatments: Better Research for Better Healthcare by Imogen Evans, Hazel Thornton and Iain Chalmers. Pinter & Martin (2010).

The Healer's Manual by Ted Andrews. Llewellyn (2005).

Quantum Healing: Exploring the Frontiers of Mind/Body Medicine by Deepak Chopra. Bantam (1990).

H is for Homeopathy

Homeopathy is the treatment of disease with minute doses of drugs that, if given in larger quantities, would cause some of the symptoms of that disease. So it is based on the idea that 'like cures like'. It aims to treat the whole body, not disconnected parts, encouraging the body to heal itself and correct imbalance. As it is non-toxic, it has no side effects.

Homeopathic hospitals exist within the National Health Service and can be found in London, Liverpool, Bristol, Glasgow and Tunbridge Wells. They offer care for a range of diseases, including cancer. But some of the ideas on which homeopathy is based do not fit well with conventional scientific thinking. For example, scientists cannot understand how it is that the more dilute a homeopathic remedy, the more powerful its effect. The explanation – that the water retains a 'memory' of the therapeutic substance – is difficult to grasp.

There are many remedies that can assist patients during radiotherapy and chemotherapy, alleviating burning and skin problems, relieving nausea, stimulating the appetite, balancing hormonal state and improving emotional problems such as depression. There are also many complex homeopathic remedies to help with detoxification after treatment and to support organs such as the liver that have been weakened. The proponents of homeopathy argue that it treats both emotional and physical states and is therefore of great benefit during conventional cancer treatments.

Further information

UK

Linda Crawford, homeopath. Email: linda@allergyline.com

British Homeopathic Association, Hahnemann House, 29 Park Street West, Luton LU1 3BE. Tel: 01582 408675. Email: info@britishhomeopathic. org. Website: www.britishhomeopathic.org

Royal London Hospital for Integrated Medicine, 60 Great Ormond Street, London WC1N 3RN. Tel: 0845 1555 000. Website: www.uclh.nhs. uk/Our+hospitals/Royal+London+Hospital+for+Integrated+Medicine. htm

Penny Brohn Cancer Care evidence-based information sheet on Homeopathy: www.pennybrohncancercare.org/upload/docs/932/homeo pathy.pdf

US

National Center for Homeopathy: www.homeopathic.org

National Center on Complementary and Alternative Medicine: http://nccam.nih.gov/health/homeopathy

References

The Memory of Water: Homeopathy and the Battle of New Ideas in the New Science by M Schiff. Thorsons (1997).

'Is evidence for homeopathy reproducible?' by D. Reilly. *The Lancet* 1994, volume 344, pages 1601–1606.

For a sceptical view, see 'The Cognitive Dissonance of Homeopathy', a short article criticizing homeopathy with references to several other good critiques at the end: http://sciencebasedpharmacy.wordpress.com/2009/01/31/the-cognitive-dissonance-of-homeopathy.

H is for Hope (Real and False)

Someone phoned me saying he had been given three months to live, with tumours in his lungs and neck which were inoperable and unlikely to respond to chemo. When I asked how he actually felt, he replied that he was fine: no pain, no suffering. So I asked if he believed that he would be dead in three months' time. He hesitated, but clearly believed what he had been told. We then discussed all the things that might make a difference to his survival, and by the end of the conversation he had found that sense of hope that had previously been quashed. A week later he telephoned to say he had decided to have injections of laetrile and vitamin C. He was optimistic and happy to be on an adventure, whatever the outcome. About three weeks later he phoned to say that the doctor who had given him such a poor prognosis had been in touch to admit to a possible wrong diagnosis. I tell this story not to draw attention to the doctor's plight (because one recognizes the difficulties and agonizing involved in his situation) but to emphasize the case for hope.

I also actually witnessed a friend's complete turnaround. He was diagnosed with bowel cancer and it was touch and go for a while. Then he was given the all-clear and had to decide what to do with the rest of his life. A crowd of us met in a pub and he talked about going back to his old job in the timber business. Some days later, I had a strong sensation that I should ring and tell him to consider something that involved use of his hands, perhaps in healing. I phoned and rather shyly told him my thoughts. He said it was strange I should ring because he had in front of him the application forms for a course in acupuncture and was considering whether or not to fill them in. 'Do it,' I said. He is now qualified, delighted with his new career, and there is no sign of any more cancer!

Another illustration of the importance of not giving up hope.

Twenty years ago, doctors practised a benign deception on many of their cancer patients. Now, it seems ingrained in their training that they must not give false hope of cure. Perhaps this teaching has floated across from America where it is designed to prevent the patient from suing the doctor if his treatment fails to 'cure'. But the explanation given is humanitarian: doctors do not want the patient to experience the deep disappointment if a treatment fails. They do not want to be responsible for patients failing to realize the truth of their situation, or to be blamed for not keeping them fully in the picture. The problem is that the doctrine of absolute truth can result in the patient abandoning hope.

Patients feeling vulnerable tend to believe their doctors' every word. The doctor, wanting to be totally honest, tells the patient that he or she only has months to live. The patient believes that, becomes despondent and starts thinking only about funerals. But hope remains.

The one-in-three risk of developing cancer at some stage in our lives applies also to the medical profession. Jerome Groopman (see 'Further information') tells the story of a professor of pathology diagnosed with stomach cancer. He knew only too well how his disease would progress to his imminent death. But he put himself through the most rigorous chemo and radiotherapy. This itself very nearly killed him, but 13 years later he was alive and free of cancer (though still having difficulty swallowing some foods). The professor had said, 'I had a crystal-clear understanding of my chances. And it was my right to choose what I did... I deeply wanted to live, so I had to fight.' Dr Groopman, who had opposed the professor's choice because of the suffering involved, commented, 'His was a libertarian mind-set, one that placed the individual squarely as the ultimate arbiter of his fate. It represented a certain form of hope – the hope to be strong enough not to yield, to have the determination and the fortitude to fight, despite knowing that there was little chance of survival.'

Dr Groopman's account tells of his recognition that 'A doctor should never write off a person a priori. At the moment of initial diagnosis, closing off options and denying choices is premature and clinically wrong.' He quotes Oliver Wendell-Holmes, a nineteenth-century physician and poet from Boston: 'Beware how you take away hope from another human being.'

Part of the remit of Penny Brohn Cancer Care (formerly Bristol Cancer Help Centre) is the transformational aspect of cancer. During my week's course there in February 2003 I met Kate. She had first been diagnosed with breast cancer, in May 1995, aged 37. In 1999 she was diagnosed with liver cancer. When I met her, she was extremely jaundiced, but in fantastic good spirits and with loads of energy. Kate encouraged me to write this book and sent me cards, the last of which was of an impenetrable castle or fortress – a strong, unwavering, uncompromising image. She wrote to me a week before she died in June 2003, leaving behind her two daughters and her husband. She wanted me to use her letter to help others. This is what she says about hope:

> *My oncologist said to me at my last appointment in April 2003 that someone who had got to my stage in my liver cancer and was as jaundiced as I was didn't last more than a few days, a week at most. I have been extremely yellow since January 2003 and it appears that I have kept myself alive and the medical profession doesn't know how. I reckon it's because I have never given up hope and still haven't although I know that my time is nearly up which I have accepted and this allows me to deal with things that others don't get a chance to because they generally don't know when they'll die. ...I feel privileged that I have been given the opportunity to have the time to talk to those I love, or write to them what I am feeling.*

In this letter, Kate explained how much support and encouragement she received from her oncologist, who was an integral part of her survival team and only too delighted that she 'baffled medical science' by surviving so well so long.

Not all oncologists are like this, of course…

I have heard a story – and story it is, although it is not beyond the realms of possibility. In order to 'deal with' NHS patients' allocated time slot of 15 minutes (he has a waiting room of 30 in an afternoon), he has a strategy worked out. The patient comes in, asks the usual questions: Must I have chemotherapy? How long have I got, doc? He says, 'You've got two years, and that's if you take the chemo and be a good girl.' She bursts into tears and is unable to communicate further. He passes her the tissues, confirms the starting date for chemo – end of interview.

This is not only callous but completely self-defeating.

The essence of the relationship between doctor and patient, as Siegel puts it, is 'the healing partnership'. In its absence, the prophecy of death becomes self-fulfilling. The opposite is shown by patients whose tumours start to shrink before their chemo and radiotherapy because the healing process begins when the doctor 'can instill some measure of hope'.

A day that stands out in my mind is the day I went to see an oncologist (not in the 'hero' category) in 2002. When he told me I had two years at most to expect, I remember thinking, 'You arrogant fellow. You are not God. This is God's decision, and God's alone.' This was a huge turning point since it started my exciting spiritual journey. So I suppose I should thank him, really. But when our paths have crossed since, I always remind him of how surprised he must be to see me!

TOP TIP
Truth and hope may sit side by side.

Further information
References

The Anatomy of Hope: How People Find Strength in the Face of Illness by Jerome Groopman. Simon and Schuster (2005).

Anatomy of the Spirit: The Seven Stages of Power and Healing by Caroline Myss. Bantam (1997).

Love, Medicine and Miracles by Bernie Siegel. Random House (1999).

H is for Hormone Replacement Therapy (HRT)

Hormones are chemicals produced by glands in one part of the body which travel in the bloodstream and have effects on organs in other parts of the body. The female hormone oestrogen, for example, is produced by the ovaries but has its main effects on the lining of the womb and breast tissue. Testosterone, produced in the testes, has effects all over the body, influencing many aspects of function, from voice quality to growth of body hair. Because breast tissue responds to oestrogen, blocking the effects of this hormone is an effective treatment for many cases of breast cancer (see 'H is for Hormone Therapy'). Similarly, prostate tissue responds to testosterone, and removing this growth stimulus is an effective treatment for prostate cancer (see 'P is for Prostate Cancer').

Also called 'chemical messengers', hormones help regulate hunger, growth, metabolic rate and our readiness for 'fight or flight'. But it is their role in the female reproductive cycle which is probably the best known.

Hormone replacement therapy (HRT) was introduced in the 1970s to treat hot flushes and night sweats suffered by women after the menopause. HRT is available in preparations that contain only oestrogen, and in a combined form in which there is both oestrogen and progesterone. HRT is very effective in relieving menopausal symptoms, although there may be side effects such as nausea and fluid retention – so it is worth trying different forms of HRT to find one that is best for you. More worryingly, there are long-term effects of HRT including an increased risk of breast, ovarian and womb cancer and of blood clots and stroke. Much has been written about this controversial area. Even though the increased risk is real, it may still be relatively small. For example, it is estimated that among a thousand 50–59-year-old women taking oestrogen-only HRT for five years, two will develop breast cancer and one will have a stroke.

Many doctors advise that taking HRT for up to five years carries an acceptable risk, given the benefits that are often experienced. But women have undoubtedly been turning to herbal alternatives and supplements to relieve menopausal symptoms. There is the usual problem of lack of scientific evidence that remedies such as black cohosh and St John's wort are effective, and the worry is that they may actually do harm, particularly if women have a medical condition such as high blood pressure. But, while the scientific evidence for efficacy might be lacking, the anecdotal evidence can be impressive. The best advice is to take a professional opinion before embarking on a course of herbal treatment or supplements. There is also the view that the menopause is simply the natural state of being for a woman of a certain age, and that a review of lifestyle, diet and exercise can be a more helpful approach than seeking treatment to reverse its effects.

Further information

UK

For information on the risks of using HRT in the development of cancer, see **Cancer Research UK**: www.cancerhelp.org.uk/about-cancer/cancer-questions/hrt-and-cancer-risk

Breakthrough Breast Cancer: http://breakthrough.org.uk/breast_cancer/breast_cancer_facts/risk_factors_general_information/hormone_replacement.html

Herbal ayurveda from **Pukka**: www.pukkaherbs.com

National Institute of Medical Herbalists, Elm House, 54 Mary Arches Street, Exeter EX4 3BA. Tel: 01392 426022. Email: info@nimh.org.uk. Website: www.nimh.org.uk

Homeopathic Medical Association, 7 Darnley Road, Gravesend, Kent DA11 0RU. Tel: 01474 560336. Email: info@the-hma.org. Website: www.the-hma.org

US

National Cancer Institute's summary of the evidence of the risks and benefits of postmenopausal use of hormones: www.cancer.gov/newscenter/archive/benchmarks-vol2-issue8/page2

Findings from the **Women's Health Initiative** (WHI) trials about HRT: www.nhlbi.nih.gov/whi

References

HRT and the Natural Alternatives by Jan Clark. Hamlyn (2003).

Breast Cancer: How Hormone Balance can Help Save Your Life by John R. Lee, David Zava and Virginia Hopkins. Grand Central Publishing (2005).

A Woman's Best Medicine for Menopause: Your Personal Guide to Radiant Good Health Using Maharishi Ayurveda by Nancy Lonsdorf. McGraw Hill (2002).

'Western herbal medicines and the menopause' by Jill Rosemary Davies. *Positive Health*, February 2004.

Hormone Heresy: What Women Must Know about their Hormones by Sherrill Sellman. Bridger House (2009).

For a critique of 'bioidentical hormone replacement', see Newsweek, 'A Blow-Up Over "Bioidenticals"': http://www.newsweek.com/2006/10/30/a-blow-up-over-bioidenticals.html.

H is for Hormone Therapy

Some tissues in the body grow in response to hormones. This is true of breast tissue in women, which responds to oestrogen and progesterone, and of prostate tissue in men, which responds to testosterone. Cancers which arise in these tissues may also be hormone-responsive. If this is the case, a logical approach to treatment is to cut off the supply of hormones.

In the case of breast cancer, histologists who examine tissue taken from the tumour will look to see if its cells express oestrogen receptors. If they do, the tumour is said to be 'ER positive' (oestrogen is 'estrogen' in the US). The cancer may also be 'PR positive', if it has progesterone receptors. Either way, it is likely that growth is being driven by hormones. So tamoxifen (which blocks oestrogen receptors) or aromatase inhibitors (which prevent oestrogen production) stand a good chance of eliminating residual disease if the cancer is caught early enough for surgery to be potentially curative. If the cancer has already spread, hormone therapy can help keep it under control, often for long periods. Breast cancer cells which do not have hormone receptors will not usually respond to hormone drugs, but they can be treated with chemotherapy.

Prostate cancer that has spread into tissues around the gland, or which has returned after radiotherapy or surgery, is generally treated with some form of hormonal therapy aimed at reducing production of testosterone or blocking its effects. Nowadays, this is usually achieved using drugs. They can be of two types: either LHRH agonists (given by injection every month or so) or anti-androgens (taken daily as tablets). Sometimes these drug treatments are combined.

An alternative approach to stopping testosterone production (though one that is now less frequently used) is to remove the testes (surgical castration, or orchidectomy). The corresponding intervention in the case of breast cancer is surgery to take out the ovaries (oophorectomy).

Further information

UK

Macmillan Cancer Support on hormonal therapies: www.macmillan. org.uk/Cancerinformation/Cancertypes/Prostate/Treatmentforearly prostatecancer/Hormonaltherapy.aspx, and www.macmillan.org.uk/Cancer information/Cancertypes/Breastsecondary/Treatingsecondarybreast cancer/Hormonaltherapies.aspx

Cancer Research UK on hormonal therapies: www.cancerhelp.org.uk/ about-cancer/treatment/hormone/what-hormone-therapy-is#Prostate, and www.cancerhelp.org.uk/about-cancer/treatment/hormone/what-hormone-therapy-is#breast

US

National Cancer Institute on hormonal therapies: www.cancer.gov/ cancertopics/pdq/treatment/breast/Patient/page5#Keypoint23, and www.cancer.gov/cancertopics/pdq/treatment/prostate/Patient/page4 #Keypoint17

EU

Professor Douwes at **Klinik St George**, Rosenheimer Str. 6–8, 83043 Bad Aibling, Germany. Tel: +011 49 8061 398 233. Website: www.klinik-st-georg.de/e/therapies/hyperthermia/index.html

Centre of Hyperthermia Practice, Siebenhüner, Vilbeler Landstrasse 45 B, 60388 Frankfurt, Germany. Website: www.hyperthermie-zentrum.de/ home.html

H is for Hyperthermia

Tumours are vulnerable to heat damage for many reasons. One is that the poor organization of their blood vessels leads to metabolic changes, and these are made more pronounced by heat. Hyperthermia, or heat treatment, is generally not used alone but to enhance the effects of other forms of treatment. Heat sensitizes cancer cells to the effects of radiation and chemotherapy. This may enable doctors to give the same dose with increased effect, or to give a lower dose (and so do less damage to healthy tissues) without losing efficacy against the cancer.

Tissue can be heated up with microwave or radiofrequency energy, or by ultrasound. Hyperthermia can be used over a small area or applied to the whole body, which is needed when a cancer has spread to other sites.

Hyperthermia is a proven treatment for inflammatory breast cancer and certain other tumours that have spread locally to the extent that they cannot be removed by surgery. A recent study by doctors in Rotterdam randomly assigned women with cancer of the cervix to treatment by radiation alone or to radiotherapy plus hyperthermia. The addition of hyperthermia almost doubled the chances of long-term survival. So results can be very impressive. For most tumours, though, the potential of hyperthermia is still being researched, and the treatment is not widely available.

Inflammatory breast cancer looks very alarming. I found it very frightening, as what looked like red welts were visibly spreading like tendrils across the surface of my right breast, creeping not that slowly to my underarm and back. This progression was literally stopped in its tracks after the first session of hyperthermia, which I had in conjunction with radiotherapy and chemotherapy using paclitaxel (Taxol) and trastuzumab (Herceptin). An applicator or 'hot plate' was gently lowered to the skin surface where the cancer had spread and heat increased to about 43°C. Treatment took a couple of hours. I had no trouble with the heat and slept through all my sessions.

Further information

US

National Cancer Institute, 'Hyperthermia in Cancer Treatment: Questions and Answers': www.cancer.gov/cancertopics/factsheet/Therapy/ hyperthermia

American Cancer Society information on hyperthermia: www.cancer.org/ Treatment/TreatmentsandSideEffects/TreatmentTypes/hyperthermia

References

'Long-term improvement in treatment outcome after radiotherapy and hyperthermia' by M. Franckena and colleagues. *International Journal of Radiation Oncology* 2008, volume 70, pages 1176–1182.

The contact for the Dutch group is M. Franckena at the Erasmus Medical Centre, Rotterdam, Email: m.franckena@erasmusmc.nl. In the UK, Dr Clare Vernon was a champion of hyperthermia when a consultant at the Hammersmith Hospital.

H is for Hypnotherapy

Hypnotherapy treats illness using hypnosis, an induced sleep-like state in which questions can be put and suggestions made. The subconscious mind is a powerful force. It always tries to protect you, and tapping into the subconscious can empower healing. It is often believed (rightly or wrongly) that cancer is 'anger turned inwards'. By releasing creative, flexible, subconscious behaviour around anger or suppressed emotions, healing can be stimulated. Hypnotherapy could also be useful for someone with cancer who is very negative about their disease and wants to try to change their outlook.

In her book on natural health, Susan Clark makes the point (see 'References' on the following page; pages 270–271) that hypnotherapy 'is a powerful tool in the right hands and a complete waste of time and money in the wrong ones'. The key is in the selection of a well-trained and experienced hypnotherapist who can really help.

If cells do communicate in a way science does not as yet understand, and it *is* possible to heal through subliminal communication, then hypnotherapy is an underused resource!

(See also 'P is for Psychoneuroimmunology and the Power of Positive Thought'.)

TOP TIP

Why not use every tool in the box?

Further information

UK

The Hypnotherapy Association, 14 Crown Street, Chorley, Lancashire PR7 1DX. Tel: 01257 262124. Email: theha@tiscali.co.uk. Website: www.thehypnotherapyassociation.co.uk

British Society of Clinical Hypnosis Tel: 01262 403103. Email: sec@bsch.org.uk. Website: www.bsch.org.uk

UK Confederation of National Hypnotherapy Organisations, Suite 404 Albany House, 324/326 Regent Street, London W1B 3HH. Tel: 0800 952 0560. Website: www.ukcho.co.uk/register-search.asp

US

National Board for Certified Clinical Hypnotherapists: www.natboard.com

American Cancer Society information on hypnosis: www.cancer.org/Treatment/TreatmentsandSideEffects/ComplementaryandAlternative Medicine/MindBodyandSpirit/hypnosis

References

'Hypnosis and Cancer: Host Defences, Quality of Life and Survival' by L.G. Walker. *Contemporary Hypnosis* 2006, volume 15, pages 34–39.

What Really Works in Natural Health by Susan Clark. Bantam (2004).

'Hypnosis before breast-cancer surgery reduces pain, discomfort, and cost': www.cancer.gov/clinicaltrials/results/summary/2007/hypnosis0907. Link to the study: http://jnci.oxfordjournals.org/cgi/content/99/17/1304.full.

I is for Immune System and Immunotherapy

The body's immune system is generally pretty effective at fighting infectious organisms that cause disease. Bacteria, for example, are recognized as clearly 'foreign' and our resources are mobilized to seek and destroy them. Many cases of cancerous change are also spotted and the malignant cells eradicated. But sometimes they avoid detection and, once a tumour begins to form, it actively secretes substances which suppress the immune response.

Immunotherapies aim to strengthen and stimulate the immune system in its fight against a cancer. Broadly, they take one of two approaches. The first is to give substances called cytokines that cause a general activation of the immune response. Examples are interferon and interleukin (see 'I is for Interleukin and Interferon'). Both are produced by the body, but both are now also available as a result of genetic engineering and so can be given as drugs. The second approach is to alert the immune system more specifically to the presence of cells from a particular kind of tumour, and sometimes even to the precise tumour present in an individual patient, in the hope that it will start to fight back. This is done by vaccination.

Tumours evolve from our normal cells and so are often seen by the immune system as 'self' and not as 'foreign', and therefore are thought not to be dangerous. As the cancer undergoes further genetic changes, it may express substances that are different from those produced by normal cells. These are called antigens. The body may recognize them and make antibodies or mount a response through the cells of the immune system. But as the cancer grows, it learns to express fewer antigens or to produce defensive agents which prevent the immune response from recognizing it. Tumours can also secrete substances that switch the immune system off.

Cancers often arise in tissues that have been inflamed for a long time. Chronic inflammation has many features of wound healing, and when a wound heals, the immune system is suppressed locally so that new repair tissue is not rejected. So chronic inflammation is an ideal environment for cancer to develop in: it can escape immune detection, as well as having lots of growth factors provided. It has recently been recognized that patients who do not respond to cancer vaccines often have signs of inflammation, which has led to the idea that they should perhaps be treated with anti-inflammatory drugs.

Immunotherapy can be targeted at antigens expressed by cancer cells, and several antibody drugs are now in regular use to fight cancer. Examples include rituximab, which targets an antigen on lymphoma cells, and trastuzumab and cetuximab, which target molecules overexpressed on breast and bowel cancers. It is interesting that all these antibodies work better when given in combination with chemotherapy.

The second approach to immunotherapy is to strengthen the anti-tumour response of immune system cells. Most important for inducing a good response are the dendritic cells: they 'present' antigens to the rest of the immune system. These cells are few and far between but can be taken from a patient's blood and reproduced in the lab with the help of growth and maturation factors. They are then exposed to pulses of tumour antigens (which may have been taken from the patient's own cancer) before being reinfused. The process has been likened to letting the bloodhounds smell an item of clothing from the person they are then sent to hunt down. The hope is that what dendritic cells learn by exposure to cancer antigens outside the body will be passed on to the rest of the immune system so that it is better able to recognize and fight the tumour.

This vaccination approach is labour-intensive and expensive. Even so, it is a major and promising line of immunotherapy research and has led to the first commercial vaccine to achieve a significant survival advantage in patients (see 'V is for Vaccines'). This was in prostate cancer, but the vaccine strategy will continue to be applied to a large number of tumours including breast cancer.

To be widely successful, though, immunotherapy will probably require a combination of approaches. For tumours that are large or have spread, it may be necessary to begin by using chemotherapy and antibodies to reduce the amount of cancer, perhaps followed by vaccination and low-dose cytokines. It is increasingly recognized that immunotherapy will be given in addition to other treatments and not instead of them.

Further information

UK

Cancer Vaccine Institute, Haysmacintyre, Fairfax House, 15 Fulwood Place, London, WC1V 6AY. Principal: Professor Angus Dalgleish, Bsc (Hons) MD FRACPath FRACP FRCP FMedSci. Website: www.cancervaccine. org.uk

US

National Cancer Institute: www.cancer.gov/cancertopics/understanding cancer/immunesystem, and www.cancer.gov/cancertopics/factsheet/Therapy/ biological

References

'Immunotherapy and the development of cancer vaccines' by A.G. Dalgleish. *Expert Review Vaccines* 2006, volume 5, pages 1–4.

'Inflammation and cancer: The role of the immune response and angiogenesis' by A.G. Dalgleish and K. O'Byrne. *Cancer Treatment Research* 2006, volume 130, pages 1–38.

I is for Interleukin and Interferon

The interleukins and interferons are members of a large family of molecules – the cytokines – that orchestrate the immune system.

Interleukin-2, a member of the family with promise in treating several kinds of cancers, causes an increase in the number of immune system cells that have been activated by recognition of an antigen. Young and fit patients who have advanced kidney cancer can be treated with high doses of interleukin-2, and this is believed to cure a small number of cases. Steven Rosenberg and his group from the US National Cancer Institute have also achieved some impressive results in a few patients with melanoma; and a recent review suggested that all patients with advanced disease who had survived long-term had had interleukin at some stage in their treatment. Recently, Rosenberg's group has been developing new techniques using the drug to increase the numbers of lymphocytes taken from patients' blood and tumours.

Interleukin was originally used in very high doses, and the side effects meant that patients had to stay in hospital for several weeks. These days it is used mostly in lower doses and given under the skin (subcutaneously) to outpatients. Low-dose interleukin-2 appears to be as effective as the high-dose regimens, especially when given in conjunction with other immunotherapies, such as vaccination, or after other kinds of treatment, such as radiotherapy, that result in death of tumour cells.

Interferon is produced when we are infected by a virus but it also has the effect of reducing cell proliferation. It has been widely investigated as a way of treating melanoma but, although it can stop the cancer progressing for a while, it does not prolong survival. And interferon is associated with severe flu-like side effects.

I is for IP6 and Inositol

Inositol (IP6) is a carbohydrate which occurs as phytic acid in large amounts in many plants including cereals, legumes and citrus fruits. Inositol is also made in our bodies and may play a role in maintaining health. Laboratory work using cancer cells grown in culture suggests that Inositol and related compounds have antioxidant properties, that they may encourage tumour cells to self-destruct and may even reverse certain of the changes that cause malignancy. But showing an effect in a laboratory dish is a long way from showing benefit in patients. That said, researchers are investigating whether IP6 can prevent precancerous abnormalities in smokers turning into lung cancer. A trial to see if Inositol can prevent development of colorectal cancer in people at high risk is planned. There is evidence from a small Croatian study in breast cancer patients that IP6/Inositol may improve quality of life and decrease the side effects of chemotherapy. But this is regarded as a pilot study, and more research is needed before the true potential of IP6 can be assessed.

Further information

UK
The original Shamsuddin formula of IP6 with Inositol is available from **Jan de Vries Healthcare**. Health Store order line: 01292 318846. Website: www.jandevrieshealth.co.uk

US
Lewis Gale Hospital website. Scroll down to 'Natural and Alternative Treatments' on the main menu and click on 'Herbs and Supplements'. Then find 'IP6' in the A–Z list: www.alleghanyregional.com/healthcontent.asp?page=contentselection/condensedmainindex

Memorial Sloan-Kettering Cancer Center: www.mskcc.org/mskcc/html/69264.cfm

References
'Protection against cancer by dietary IP6 and Inositol' by I. Vucenik and A.M. Shamsuddin. *Nutrition and Cancer* 2006, volume 55, pages 109–125.

'Efficacy of IP6+Inositol in the treatment of breast cancer patients receiving chemotherapy: Prospective, randomized, pilot clinical study' by Ivan Bacic and colleagues. *Journal of Experimental Clinical Cancer Research* 2010, volume 29.

IP6: Nature's Revolutionary Cancer-Fighter by A.M. Shamsuddin. Kensington (1998).

I is for Iscador

See 'M is for Mistletoe'

J is for Journey

Many people with cancer refer to – and feel as if they are on – a form of journey. Sometimes the phrase 'the cancer journey' is used. Certainly, cancer is a life experience, and with any experience comes learning, greater wisdom and understanding. This is why I believe cancer is not necessarily a negative incident in our lives. But it does stop us in our tracks, resulting in a reassessment of values.

As we still cannot fully explain how and why we get cancer, there is generally an appraisal of lifestyle. What is 'wrong' with our life tends to get linked in with 'the reason why' we contracted the disease. Theories range from fast foods that overload our systems with toxins, through the growth hormones passed on to us in beef and milk, to the memory contained in our cells from the moments of conception or birth. The positive aspect of this reappraisal is that we unpack what is going on in our lives. We stop and think, and from that position make choices we might not otherwise have made.

It gives us the excuse to refuse to do the things we do not want to (but feel we 'have' to do) and a reason to do the things we want. This is not to say we become totally irresponsible, just that we can examine *why* we think we should do those things we hate. If life threatens to come to an end sooner rather than later, it concentrates the mind. Do the things you want to – visit Egypt, climb a mountain in Scotland, spend time on a boat, walk in the country. Take the opportunity!

The physical journey of cancer usually involves diagnosis, surgery, chemotherapy and/or radiotherapy (though not always in that order). The mental journey is often shock upon diagnosis, stoicism and bravery in the face of adversity, then coming to terms with living with cancer and, in some cases, coming to terms with dying of it. The spiritual journey can be extremely exciting. Cancer is sometimes referred to as a 'wake-up' call. It was in my case. On diagnosis or shortly after, I realized my spirit had certainly awakened and was reporting for duty. In making choices, my spirit was right there. I started to see my life in context. Everything that I had ever done or experienced had brought me to this one point. I did not know whether I would live or die, but I found an inner peace in accord with whichever outcome.

TOP TIP

Whilst cancer might seem the big bad black cloud, have you checked for the silver lining?

Further information

References

The Journey: An Extraordinary Guide for Healing Your Life and Setting Yourself Free by Brandon Bays. Element Harper Collins (2003).

The Healing Journey: Overcoming the Crisis of Cancer by Alastair J. Cunningham. Key Healing Journey Books (2010).

A Visible Wound: A Healing Journey through Breast Cancer by Julie Friedeberger. Element Books (1996).

Happiness in a Storm: Facing Illness and Embracing Life as a Healthy Survivor by Wendy S. Harpham. W.W. Norton and Co. (2005).

J is for Juicing

Research during the past few decades suggests the anti-cancer properties of a diet low in fat and animal protein and high in whole grains and fibre, fruit and vegetables (see also the Bristol Approach to Healthy Eating in 'P is for Penny Brohn Cancer Care'). Plants incorporate minerals from the soil, so fruits and vegetables provide an excellent source of nutrients. Some people suggest that by separating the minerals from some of the plant fibre, juicing may release them in a more bio-available form, facilitating efficient absorption and reducing strain on the digestive system.

Improving and maintaining anti-cancer protection within the cells is vital when fighting the disease. The immune system's ability to recognize and destroy abnormal cells depends on many factors including the hormonal, emotional and nutritional. By providing the body with a rich source of vitamins, minerals, live enzymes, amino acids and a vast array of phytochemicals, the hope is that fresh juices can help maintain this frontline defence. They may also assist in detoxifying the body, protecting it from the effects both of the cancer and of medical treatment while enhancing the efficacy of conventional medicine.

Excellent for juicing are leafy, green cruciferous vegetables such as broccoli, cabbage, watercress, kale and bok choy which are rich in minerals, especially calcium, and in folates (see 'F is for Folic Acid'). It is believed that the chlorophyll content of the vegetable has a cleansing and healing effect on the digestive tract and liver.

Also powerfully antioxidant are the carrot family of fruits and vegetables. Rich in beta-carotene (the precursor to vitamin A) and vitamin C, spinach, sweet potatoes, carrots, beetroot, green and red bell peppers, apricots, peaches, papaya and lemons are good sources. Considered over the last few years as being more powerful a protective antioxidant than vitamin A and beta-carotene, lycopene can be found in tomatoes, watermelon and pink grapefruit. Tomatoes processed by heating have the highest amounts of lycopene, so you might add a can of tomatoes to your favourite juice!

Although perhaps not an obvious choice for juicing, onions and garlic (see 'G is for Garlic') both contain allicin, a sulphur compound required by the liver for effective detoxification. Juiced with carrots and digestive-tract-cleansing apples – a good sweetening basis for any juice – their strong flavour can be disguised!

By law, commercially made fruit and vegetable juices have to be pasteurized. The heating required destroys the health-giving plant enzymes, so it is much better to make your own juice. Where possible, choose fresh, local, organic produce that is in season.

Many nutrients are just below the skin of fruit and vegetables and can be lost on peeling. Soaking in a weak solution of water and apple cider vinegar or washing in dilute biodegradable washing-up liquid will ensure that pesticides are removed. Sometimes a light scrub may be needed before rinsing in clear water and juicing.

There are many juicers available (see 'Further information' below). Choosing one with a wide feed tube saves time since it avoids the need to cut the produce into small pieces. Centrifugal extractors are popular and well priced. Masticating juicers, in particular those with twin gears, use a slow-speed extraction process to prevent oxygenation of the juice. It can then be stored for up to 48 hours. Reviews indicate that the juice delivered is of the highest quality in terms of vitamin, mineral and live enzyme content.

TOP TIP

It may not always be practical to drink the juice immediately after preparation. Adding a teaspoon of vitamin C powder or a squeeze of lemon to the base of the juicing jug acts as an antioxidant, preventing the juice from turning brown. Cover and store in the fridge or thermos flask for a nutritious, uplifting drink during the day. The residual fibre can be used to thicken soups or, failing that, makes very good compost!

Further information
UK
For reviews, best buy suggestions and stockists see **Which?**: www.which.co.uk/juicers

For juicers and juicing books see **UK Juicers**: www.ukjuicers.com, and **Juiceland**: www.juiceland.co.uk

US
Juicer reviews from **Consumersearch**: www.consumersearch.com/juicers

Some recipes from **ZestyCook**: http://zestycook.com/the-power-of-juice-juicer-recipes

References
Superjuice: Juicing for Health and Healing by Michael Van Straten. Mitchell Beazley (1999).

The Top 100 Juices: 100 Juices to Turbo-charge Your Body with Vitamins and Minerals by Sarah Owen. Duncan Baird (2007).

The Big Book of Juices and Smoothies: 365 Natural Blends for Health and Vitality Every Day by Natalie Savona. Duncan Baird (2003).

The Rainbow Diet - and How It Can Help You Beat Cancer by Chris Woollams (2010). Order from www.canceractive.com.

New Optimum Nutrition Bible by Patrick Holford. Crossing Press (2005).

What to Eat if You Have Cancer (Revised): Healing Foods that Boost Your Immune System by Maureen Keane and Daniella Chace. McGraw-Hill Contemporary (2006).

Juice Lady's Guide to Juicing for Health: Unleashing the Healing Power of Whole Fruits and Vegetables by Cherie Calbom. Avery Press/Penguin Putnam (2009).

L is for Laetrile (and Apricot Kernels)

Laetrile, which is also called vitamin B17 (though some say is not a vitamin at all) is a synthetic version of a substance (amygdalin) that occurs naturally in certain nuts, such as almonds, and fruits – and particularly in the kernels of apricots. Whether laetrile or apricot kernels can help cancer patients is a highly contentious issue. Most doctors practising conventional medicine think that these substances have no beneficial effects and can in fact do harm (because they may release cyanide). Enthusiasts argue that there is a good rationale for their use against cancer and that failure to acknowledge this amounts to a conspiracy among doctors and drug companies.

Part of the argument for laetrile is that our modern diet lacks natural sources of B17 (found, for example, in millet) and that cancer is, in essence, due to B17 deficiency. It is claimed that certain remote peoples, such as the Hunza in the Himalayas, do not suffer from cancer because they have a diet high in B17 – in the case of the Hunza this is derived mostly from apricot kernels. If you accept these arguments, then treating cancer with a good source of B17 is logical. The case is made extensively in the website at www.anticancerinfo.co.uk/b17-food.htm. There appears to be some evidence of an anti-cancer effect using B17 in laboratory animals, but it is quite common for agents effective in the laboratory to be ineffective in patients. There are anecdotal reports that cancer patients have been helped, but the only trial to look systematically at the effects of laetrile (in 175 patients) found no evidence that it worked.

Laetrile is not authorized for sale in the European Union and is banned in the United States by the Food and Drug Administration. The FDA has prosecuted those selling the agent. How can this be explained?

Some suggest that the cure for cancer is being actively suppressed by a near-universal conspiracy in which the pharmaceutical industry and an equally venal medical profession are unholy partners. There is no doubt that doctors and drug companies sometimes have financial interests in common and that these shared interests have often gone undisclosed. But it would be hard to argue that doctors in general are willing to see their patients die just to line their own pockets. And doctors don't seem to use laetrile to treat themselves or their relatives who have cancer.

Besides, for every medical interest keen to promote expensive cancer drugs, there are governments and taxpayer-funded agencies desperate to see the most effective treatments available at the lowest cost. If the answer to every cancer was a B17 injection or a diet of apricots, they would be delighted.

The Cancer Research UK website is very sceptical about the value of laetrile. Follow the links from 'Types of treatment' to 'Complementary and alternative therapies', and then 'Information on individual therapies'.

Note that in 2006 the Food Standards Agency in the UK issued a warning about the possible risk to health from excessive consumption of bitter apricot kernels. They were worried about the cyanide content and advised that a safe intake would be no more than two kernels a day or their equivalent.

TOP TIPS

There is indeed a very bitter taste to an apricot kernel, so it helps to have a small cube of Green & Black's Organic Darker Shade of Milk Chocolate to hand. After meals this combination is simply delicious. An apricot kernel also goes extremely well with dates.

My tip for breakfast is to grind the kernels and sprinkle them over porridge or muesli with fresh fruit, soya yoghurt, organic honey or maple syrup.

Further information
US

National Cancer Institute's Physician Data Query (PDQ) on laetrile: www.cancer.gov/cancertopics/pdq/cam/laetrile/patient

American Cancer Society on laetrile: www.cancer.org/Treatment/ TreatmentsandSideEffects/ComplementaryandAlternativeMedicine/ PharmacologicalandBiologicalTreatment/laetrile

Memorial Sloan-Kettering Cancer Center on laetrile: www.mskcc.org/mskcc/html/69118.cfm

References

World without Cancer: The story of Vitamin B17 by G. Edward Griffin. American Media (CA) (2010).

New Cancer Therapies: The Patient's Dilemma by Penelope Williams. Firefly (2000); particularly pages 135–140.

The Cancer Industry: The Classic Exposé on the Cancer Establishment (New Updated Edition) by Ralph Moss. Equinox Press (1996); chapters 8 and 9.

Cancer: Why We're Still Dying to Know the Truth by Philip Day. Credence (1999).

For a sceptical review of laetrile's history, see 'The Rise and Fall of Laetrile' at *Quackwatch*: www.quackwatch.org/01QuackeryRelatedTopics/Cancer/laetrile.html.

L is for Laser Therapy

In laser therapy, the heat energy of a hugely amplified and precisely directed beam of light burns away cancerous tissue. In essence, this is a form of surgery, with the intense light beam acting as a cutting tool, much like a scalpel. Laser therapy can be used to restore the ability to swallow in patients with cancer of the oesophagus, and to relieve breathlessness when a tumour blocks one of the larger airways in the lung. The laser beam is channelled to where it is needed through a fibreoptic cable threaded through a flexible tube (or endoscope).

Laser treatment has several advantages. First, it seals (cauterizes) blood vessels as it cuts through them, so there is less bleeding than with conventional surgery. Second, unlike radiotherapy – which slows tumour growth but can generally only be given once to the same site in the body – laser treatment can be repeated as often as it is needed. Lasers can also be used to remove cancers of the skin, and precancerous cells on the cervix. Laser procedures have few side effects and can often be carried out on an outpatient basis.

Further information

UK

National Medical Laser Centre at University College London, 1st Floor, Charles Bell House, 67–73 Riding House Street, London W1W 7EJ. Tel: 020 7679 9060. Email: med.laser@ucl.ac.uk. Website: www.ucl.ac.uk/surgicalscience/departments_research/gsrg/nmlc

US

National Cancer Institute information on laser therapy: www.cancer.gov/cancertopics/factsheet/Therapy/lasers

American Cancer Society information on laser therapy for cancer: www.cancer.org/Treatment/TreatmentsandSideEffects/TreatmentTypes/lasers-in-cancer-treatment

Robert Wood Johnson University Hospital on laser therapy for cancer treatment: www.rwjuh.edu/health_information/centers_cancer_lasrthr.html

L is for Leukaemia

See also 'L is for Lymphoma'

Leukaemia is a cancer of white blood cells. The term derives from the Greek words *leukos* for 'white' and *haima* for 'blood'. (It is because of the word *haima* that the study of blood and its disorders is called haematology.)

Blood is produced in our bone marrow. From it come three blood components: the platelets involved in blood clotting, the red cells that carry oxygen, and the white cells that recognize invading organisms and fight infection. All of these cells have a very limited life (about three days in the case of white cells), which means that the marrow is constantly having to replace blood components. With such emphasis on rapid cell division, it is perhaps not surprising that the marrow's production of cells sometimes becomes out of control.

We speak of white cells as if they are all of the same type. In fact, there are dozens of different kinds, each with a specialized role in defending the body. Mature white cells derive from less specialized progenitors which, in turn, arise from a single type of ancestor or 'stem cell'. The plant analogy is appropriate: we have, in effect, a common stem from which branches fork, dividing again and again. At each dividing point, the cells produced are more specialized in form and function.

Blood Cell Development

Mature blood cells develop along branching lines of specialisation from their progenitors in the bone marrow. Cancerous changes can arise at any point. This accounts for the many different lymphomas and leukaemias that occur.

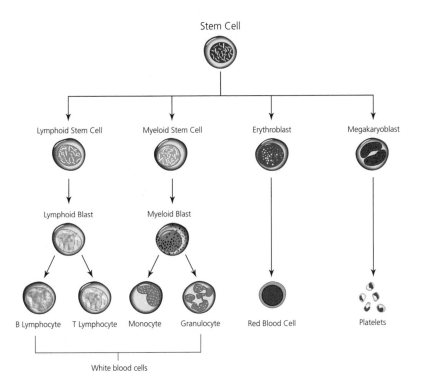

Stem Cell

Lymphoid Stem Cell   Myeloid Stem Cell   Erythroblast   Megakaryoblast

Lymphoid Blast   Myeloid Blast

B Lymphocyte   T Lymphocyte   Monocyte   Granulocyte   Red Blood Cell   Platelets

White blood cells

Because the strict controls governing cell division can break down at any stage along the branching paths of cell development, there is the potential for many different kinds of leukaemia. Some arise early in the process of specialization, and so produce large numbers of cells that are relatively primitive. Others occur at later stages along the pathways towards specialization, in which case the cells that are overproduced are more mature.

The characteristics of the leukaemia, and how it is best treated, depend on the stage at which the cancerous change occurs. But, wherever that was, excess white cells eventually spill out from the bone marrow into circulating blood where they can easily be detected.

The cancerous white cells also overwhelm healthy blood-forming cells within the marrow, interfering with the production of normal white and red cells and platelets. So we have a series of potential problems: too many immature white cells that are not fit to fight infection, a dearth of oxygen carrying red cells (i.e. anaemia), and a lack of platelets to stop bleeding.

Treatment that reduces the number of abnormal white cells in circulation can relieve symptoms. But, to achieve a cure, we have to eradicate the cell that became malignant in the first place. If this cell lies far back along the branching lines of development, close to the stem, we have to use drugs to wipe out most (or all) of the blood-forming system. And then the marrow has to be replaced with healthy cells through transplantation. These cells can come either from a donor or (before chemotherapy is given) from patients themselves. If the marrow comes from patients, it has to be cleared of cancer cells before it is reinfused. Fifteen years ago, most such transplants involved marrow taken from the hollow core of the bones themselves (usually in the hip). Nowadays the transplant is more likely to use stem cells harvested from blood.

Although there is a huge number of subtypes, leukaemias are considered as falling into four main groups. The classification is based on whether the onset of the disease was sudden or gradual (i.e. *acute* or *chronic*) and according to the broad category of white cell from which the disease arose.

So leukaemias are either *myeloid* (meaning that they developed from the cells that give rise to the monocytes and granulocytes) or *lymphocytic* (meaning that they arose from the uncontrolled growth of one of the lymphoid cells that produce B or T lymphocytes).

Acute myeloid leukaemia (AML) occurs mostly in adults. Examination of blood under the microscope shows an excess of large and immature ('poorly differentiated') cells – which doctors term 'blasts' – that form at an early stage in the development of white cells. Modern drug treatment now succeeds in controlling the disease, leading in many cases to long periods of remission. However, AML tends to recur and require further treatment. At this stage, doctors may recommend intensive chemotherapy followed by a bone marrow or stem cell transplant.

Acute lymphocytic leukaemia (ALL) is generally a disease of children. It used to be rapidly fatal, but more than 80% of cases are now cured by intensive chemotherapy.

Chronic myeloid leukaemia (CML) develops not from primitive and rapidly growing blast cells, as in the acute form of the disease, but from well-differentiated cells almost indistinguishable from their healthy counterparts. The disease is slow to make itself felt and, in its early stages, relatively harmless. But – after several years – the stem cells in the marrow switch from producing mature myeloid cells to producing cells of the kind seen in acute myeloid leukaemia. This transformation (termed 'blast crisis') moves the patient into an accelerated form of the disease.

Examining the nucleus of CML cells shows that there has been a specific translocation of genetic material: part of chromosome 9 is missing from its usual position and appears instead attached to chromosome 22. This causes the cell to produce an abnormal protein that acts as a growth signal. Ten years ago, doctors started to give CML patients a drug designed specifically to block this growth signal. The drug (imatinib) very effectively prevents the disease from progressing to blast crisis and has saved many lives.

Chronic lymphocytic leukaemia (CLL) typically occurs in the elderly. It is a relatively benign cancer in the sense that the disease usually progresses slowly. Many people live with few problems other than the need to visit the doctor regularly to have their blood count checked. If the disease starts to cause symptoms (perhaps because of swollen lymph nodes or spleen), it can be treated with chemotherapy drugs such as fludarabine, cyclophosphamide or chlorambucil. In a fit person who needs more intensive treatment, a stem cell transplant is an option.

So too is additional drug treatment with the more recently developed, targeted antibody agents rituximab (Rituxan) and alemtuzumab (Campath).

Further information

UK

Cancer Research UK: www.cancerhelp.org.uk/type/leukaemia/?script =true

Macmillan Cancer Support: www.macmillan.org.uk/Cancerinformation/ cancertypes/Leukaemia/Leukaemiaoverview.aspx

US

National Cancer Institute: www.cancer.gov/cancertopics/types/leukemia

The Leukemia and Lymphoma Society: www.leukemia-lymphoma.org/ hm_lls

L is for Life

How do you value life? What is the nature of life? These are key questions. But even more key is the question of whether you would ever have thought of asking them if you had not been diagnosed with cancer.

The diagnosis raises fundamental issues we should all be facing – if only our careers, the laundry, housework, having fun, or even reading the newspapers or watching TV had not had priority. These are difficult questions and there is no real pressure to answer them. The sheer pace of life does not give us the time. *Unless*, of course, your life is threatened.

I have mentioned how empowering a diagnosis of cancer can be. It gives you the power to say, 'I am not doing household chores this morning, I am going to the library to find out what I can about life.' And is it a problem if the children come home from school and today's lesson is how to pick their clothes up off the floor, divide them into whites and coloureds, place them in the washing machine, and turn it on? My godson, aged four, is a wizard at synchronizing the DVD and TV, and pretty impressive on GameBoy. Turning on the washing machine would literally be child's play.

There has been a 'thrill' about life this week. A deep snowfall, children (and adults) playing in it, and the sense of wonder and joy as snowpersons stand to attention across the land and townscapes. The challenge of keeping the roads clear and safe and the railways running has brought out our best.

And I remember the absolute beauty of dew on a rose, of a warm summer's day, of breeze in the sails, of a fresh tomato sandwich, of tramping through the coloured leaves and the smell of autumn – all these I love and value. (You will have your own list!) And how much more do I love and value them when I consider the possibility of never experiencing these things again. The senses of smell, touch, sight, hearing (the birds' spring chatter at 3 a.m. – even in the centre of London) and taste (not good at the moment – rather metallic!) take on an extraordinary importance. This physicality in the visible world is in direct contrast with the ephemeral, non-physical, non-visible spiritual world. Both the visible and the non-visible make up God's world.

There are people whom I love so, so much. When I consider I might be leaving them, I think I am actually only going to be in the next room. I seem to know we will all be together, part of a collective consciousness. So I have learnt to value this time on earth and the special people who surround me.

In Britain, the seasons remind us of the cyclical nature of life: the winter sleep, the bursting into life and energy of spring, basking in the glory of summer, the autumnal reflection of a world making ready to sleep again. Perhaps to understand that is to understand the journey of our souls, from the physical presence to the ephemeral being.

TOP TIP

Value every minute in joy.

Further information

Reference

Living Magically: A New Vision of Reality by Gill Edward. Piatkus (2009).

L is for Lumpectomy

If it has been established that a breast lump is malignant (see 'B is for Biopsy') but still relatively small, it can be removed along with an area of tissue around it. This procedure is sometimes called a wide local excision but is more generally known as a lumpectomy. The surrounding tissue will be examined under a microscope to see if it contains any cancer cells. If its edges (or 'margins') are clear of such cells, it is likely that no further surgery is required. But it will be necessary to have radiotherapy to the area of the breast, in an effort to make doubly sure that no cancer cells survive. Research has shown that breast-conserving surgery followed by radiation is as effective as removal of the whole breast (mastectomy) when the cancer is small and shows no signs of having spread. If, on the other hand, there are cancer cells in the margin of the removed tissue, further surgery – and perhaps a mastectomy – may be required.

Lumpectomies can also be carried out as a means of establishing the diagnosis. If this is the aim of surgery, the lump is removed initially without any surrounding tissue. If examination in the lab (see 'H is for Histology') shows that the lump is in fact a cancer, it is likely that a second operation will be needed.

Further information
UK
Breakthrough Breast Cancer: www.breakthrough.org.uk/breast_cancer/treatment/lumpectomy.html

US
Breastcancer.org: www.breastcancer.org
Imaginis: www.imaginis.com/breast-health/lumpectomy-2

L is for Lung Cancer

In men, lung cancer is second only to prostate cancer in the frequency with which it occurs; among women, it is the most common cancer after that of the breast. In both sexes, lung cancer is the tumour most likely to prove fatal. In the UK, lung cancer causes around 35,000 deaths every year. In the US, almost 160,000 people die each year from the disease. And there is a sad irony here because around 90% of cases are caused by smoking and so are preventable.

One encouraging fact is that the death rate from lung cancer among men has been falling steadily since the 1980s, as they started to quit smoking. Among women, who adopted the habit more recently and have not given up in such large numbers, the best that can be said is that the death toll exacted by the disease has now stopped increasing. The risk of lung cancer begins to fall almost as soon as a person gives up and after 10–15 years is back to the low level of a non-smoker. As well as lung cancer, smoking causes tumours of the larynx, trachea and bladder, and it is a major contributor to heart disease.

While smoking is by far the most important cause, there are, of course, other risk factors for lung cancer. Perhaps the most important are exposure to other people's smoke ('passive smoking') and occupational exposure to asbestos and diesel fumes. Radioactive radon gas seeping into houses from rocks such as granite in the ground below also plays a part.

As with all tumours, if lung cancer is caught at an early enough stage – before it has spread locally to lymph nodes or to distant parts of the body – the disease can be cured. Surgery is the mainstay of curative treatment, and an operation may remove part or all of the affected lung. High doses of radiation (radical radiotherapy) can also contribute to the cure of small tumours. The use of radiofrequency ablation (destruction) of small tumours is a new technique that holds promise.

But most cases of lung cancer are difficult to treat successfully, for several reasons. First, the disease is often quite advanced before it is diagnosed. We do not yet have an effective means of screening, and the most frequent symptoms such as cough, shortness of breath and chest pain are associated with a wide range of conditions. With lung cancer, symptoms do not generally occur until the tumour is quite large, and by this time it may already have seeded secondary cancers in other organs.

If this has happened, treating the lung tumour itself by surgery and radiotherapy will not cure the disease. A second reason is that most cases of lung cancer occur in the elderly (the peak age for diagnosis is 70–85 years). After a lifetime smoking, many older people with lung cancer are not fit enough to tolerate major surgery because they have cardiovascular or other lung problems such as chronic obstructive pulmonary disease (chronic bronchitis and emphysema).

Most lung cancers are not very sensitive to chemotherapy, but around 20% are of the 'small cell' type. This kind of lung cancer tends to spread quickly (making surgery less of an option), but it does frequently respond to drug treatment. Chemotherapy regimens usually involve combinations of two or more of the following drugs: ifosfamide, cisplatin or carboplatin, etoposide, vincristine, gemcitabine and paclitaxel. Chemotherapy can keep small-cell lung cancer under control for a while. It almost always starts to regrow, but can be treated again with a drug such as doxorubicin or, in less fit patients, topotecan.

Cancers which are not of the 'small cell' type account for the majority of lung tumours and respond less well to chemotherapy. Even so, such treatment can improve symptoms and prolong life. Options include docetaxel or paclitaxel, cisplatin or carboplatin, gemcitabine and vinorelbine. There may also be help from drugs that block proteins in or around the tumour cell that encourage cancers to grow or develop their own blood supply. New agents that have proved effective in non-small-cell lung cancer include erlotinib and cetuximab, which block a growth factor, and bevacizumab, which reduces a tumour's ability to develop its own blood vessels (see 'D is for Drugs').

Further information
UK

Cancer Research UK: www.cancerhelp.org.uk/type/lung-cancer/?script=true

Macmillan Cancer Support: www.macmillan.org.uk/Cancerinformation/cancertypes/Lung/Lungcancer.aspx

US
National Lung Cancer Partnership: www.nationallungcancerpartnership. org

National Cancer Institute: www.cancer.gov/cancertopics/types/lung

Lung Cancer Alliance, a national non-profit organization dedicated to patient support and advocacy for people living with lung cancer and those at risk of the disease: www.lungcanceralliance.org

L is for Lymphatic System

We are familiar with the circulation of the blood through arteries and veins. We are far less familiar with a system of vessels which conducts another fluid – the colourless lymph – throughout the body. Because there is no dramatic pump at the heart of it to drive the system, because the lymph channels are mostly too small to see with the naked eye, and because the function of the whole set-up (at first sight) is rather mysterious, we live largely in ignorance of its importance in health and disease.

One function of the lymphatic system is to allow white cells to travel to and from the lymph nodes (which we sometimes call glands) where they recognize foreign organisms or abnormal cells and, if needed, generate a local immune response. When these nodes swell because we have an infection, we become aware of them in the armpit, neck or groin. Indeed, the enlarged nodes may be very painful. But there are also lymph nodes, many of them too deep to feel, around the intestine and the lungs and spread throughout the body.

The lymph vessels also have a second function. Most of the watery fluid that seeps out of the blood capillaries to bathe the cells of the body is collected by tiny veins. But some collects in the lymph vessels and is pushed along by the contraction of skeletal muscles until it rejoins the blood circulation through lymph ducts that drain into veins close to the heart.

There are certain cancers called lymphomas (see 'L is for Lymphoma') in which malignant white cells accumulate in the lymph nodes causing abnormal enlargement. And cancers that have formed in any organ such as the breast, lung or colon may seed cells that travel along the lymph channels and lodge in lymph nodes. For this reason, doctors may want to take out lymph nodes and look at them under the microscope to see if they contain cancer cells.

If a lymph node is blocked by cancer, or if part of the lymph system is removed during surgery, lymph fluid can no longer drain away as it should but accumulates and causes swelling known as lymphoedema. This problem most frequently affects an arm or leg. It can be helped by raising the affected limb, compression garments and gentle massage to promote flow of lymph away from the swollen area (see 'M is for Massage').

Further information

UK

Lymphoedema Support Network, St Luke's Crypt, Sydney Street, London SW3 6NH. Tel: 020 7351 0990. Website: www.lymphoedema.org

US

National Lymphedema Network (information on lymphedema and resources for treatment): www.lymphnet.org/resourceGuide/findTreatment.htm

L is for Lymphoma

Like leukaemias, lymphomas are cancers caused by white cells dividing out of control. When the malignant cells are mostly circulating in the blood, the problem is leukaemia. When the cancer is confined mostly to the lymph glands, we call them lymphomas. Certain differences on the surface of the cancer cells influence whether they are likely to spread out and circulate or clump together in the nodes.

The swollen glands in our necks when we have a sore throat return to normal size when the infection resolves and we do not need extra white cells to fight it. Lymph nodes that become enlarged because of a lymphoma continue to grow. There may also be symptoms such as weight loss, unexplained fevers and (particularly) night sweats. But the only way to be certain of the diagnosis is to remove one of the abnormal lymph nodes and examine it under a microscope.

Because there are dozens of different kinds of lymphocyte, there are dozens of different types of lymphoma. One that stands out from the rest is called Hodgkin's disease (or Hodgkin's lymphoma). This occurs mostly in young adults and can be cured in 80% or more of cases. Most patients are treated with a combination of chemotherapy drugs (such as doxorubicin, bleomycin, vinblastine, dacarbazine) and radiotherapy to the part of the body (usually the chest) where there are swollen lymph nodes. If the disease does not respond to treatment or recurs after a period of remission, it is usual for patients to be offered a marrow or stem cell transplant.

Other types of lymphoma (reasonably enough) are called non-Hodgkin's lymphoma (or NHL). But this umbrella term covers diseases which have hugely different characters. Some (called low-grade, or indolent) progress only slowly, while others follow an aggressive course. The more aggressive lymphomas respond well to combination chemotherapy but tend to recur. Adding the antibody drug rituximab (Rituxan) to chemotherapy significantly prolongs survival.

Further information
UK

Lymphoma Association: http://www.lymphomas.org.uk

Cancer Research UK: www.cancerhelp.org.uk/type/lymphoma/?script =true

Macmillan Cancer Support: www.macmillan.org.uk/Cancerinformation/ Cancertypes/Lymphoma/Lymphomaoverview.aspx

US

National Cancer Institute information on Hodgkin's lymphoma: www. cancer.gov/cancertopics/types/hodgkin

National Cancer Institute information on non-Hodgkin's lymphoma: www.cancer.gov/cancertopics/types/non-hodgkin

Lymphoma Research Foundation: www.lymphoma.org

Patients Against Lymphoma: www.lymphomation.org

A
B
C
D
E
F
G
H
I
J
K
L

M

N
O
P
Q
R
S
T
U
V
W
X
Y
Z

M is for Macmillan Cancer Support

In 1911, a young man named Douglas Macmillan watched his father die from cancer. Intensely moved by his father's suffering, he founded the Society for the Prevention and Relief of Cancer. His objective was to provide information and support, homes for patients at low cost and voluntary nurses to attend to patients in their own homes. Much of Douglas's legacy lives on. Macmillan Cancer Support continues to be a source of support for people living with cancer and is a force in improving care.

In 2008, Macmillan merged with Cancerbackup, then the UK's leading cancer information charity and provider of award-winning publications and a specialist nurse helpline. This helpline joined with Macmillan's Cancer and Benefits helplines in 2009 to form an integrated service. By calling one number (0808 808 00 00) people can receive emotional, practical and financial support or simply chat about their concerns or ask any question about cancer.

Macmillan also launched a new website offering information about cancers and treatments, details of free publications and support services, and featuring the UK's largest online cancer community. This is where people can talk to each other about their experiences and share advice and tips. Also on the website is Macmillan's Cancer Voices Network which lists opportunities for patients to work with health and social care professionals to shape the future of cancer care. Opportunities include attending events or conferences, giving media interviews and contributing to research.

Macmillan actively campaigns for improved cancer care. Successful in its prescription charges campaign – so that people with cancer are now entitled to free prescriptions – Macmillan is currently campaigning for England to come into line with the rest of the UK and offer free or reduced-cost hospital car parking for people with cancer. It is also calling on the government and energy companies to support people with cancer who are struggling to cope with rising fuel bills.

Macmillan aims to offer practical and emotional support from the moment of diagnosis. The charity's website provides information about treatments, side effects, supportive or complementary therapies which may help alleviate the symptoms of cancer and improve quality of life, and guidance on applying for benefits to which a person with cancer or their carer may be entitled. The organization also provides grants that may help pay for heating bills, travel costs to hospital or household items such as washing machines. Macmillan recently launched the Macmillan Quality Environment Mark which is awarded to hospitals, hospices and care homes that meet standards of accessibility, privacy and dignity compiled with the help of people living with cancer.

Historically associated mainly with palliative care, Macmillan nurses now provide support from the point of diagnosis. Should a patient have an advanced cancer and require nursing at home, a palliative care team of specialist nurses can be directly involved. Macmillan nurses visit the patient and form a link between the home and local community and medical services. Specializing in pain management, symptom control, counselling and emotional support for patients and their families, the services of Macmillan nurses are free and their role is vital in helping patients die at home if that is what they want to do.

TOP TIP

Macmillan is an extensive resource helping people with cancer, their family and friends in making informed choices with professional support. It provides a great deal more than end-of-life care.

Further information
UK
Macmillan Cancer Support, 89 Albert Embankment, London SE1 7UQ. Tel: 0808 808 0000. Website: www.macmillan.org.uk

M is for Maggie's Centres

Maggie Jenks was diagnosed with cancer, staggered out of the consultant's door in complete shock and into a hostile hospital corridor. She had not been expecting this diagnosis and, even if she had, she maintained that nothing would have prepared her for it. Standing there, not knowing what to do next, she vowed that other women would be helped to avoid her situation. And the idea of the Maggie's Centres, which are spreading through the UK, was born. Her philosophy is that anyone diagnosed with cancer needs special consideration, special help and special support.

The Centres offer the chance to sit, talk, obtain information and take part in relaxation and other classes – all in a specially designed, light, airy, non-institutional setting which requires no appointments and no payment. Under one roof, you can access help with information, benefits advice, psychological support both individually and in groups, courses and stress-reducing strategies. They are there for anybody who feels the need for help, which includes those who love and look after someone with cancer.

Maggie was a landscape designer as well as an architect, and gardens are an important element of her centres. The first Maggie's Centre opened in Edinburgh in 1996. There are now centres in Glasgow, Dundee, the Highlands, Fife and London, and interim centres in Oxford, south-west Wales, Lanarkshire and Hong Kong. Centres are planned for Nottingham, the North East, the Cotswolds, Aberdeen and Barcelona. The UK centres are part of National Health Service cancer hospitals.

TOP TIP

If you have a Maggie's Centre in your area, this is the place to go; and if you do not, you can be part of the team to make it happen.

Further information

UK

Maggie's Centres, 8 Newton Place, Glasgow G3 7PR. Tel: 0300 123 1801. Email: enquiries@maggiescentres.org. Website: www.maggiescentres. org

US

Gilda's Club is a similar organization with the aim of creating welcoming communities of free support for everyone living with cancer along with their families and friends. They complement medical care by providing networking and support groups, workshops, education and social activities. The organization is named after Gilda Radner, a comedian who died from ovarian cancer: www.gildasclub.org

The Wellness Community, which also offers support and educational programmes for cancer patients and their families, is in the process of merging with Gilda's Club: www.thewellnesscommunity.org

M is for Mammogram

Mammography is a procedure in which low-dose X-rays are used to screen women for breast cancer. Each breast is carefully compressed and then one or more X-ray views are taken. In Britain, women aged between 50 and 70 years are routinely called for screening every three years. Women who are at particular risk of breast cancer may have mammography more frequently and starting at a younger age.

The technique can detect cancers that are too small to be felt as lumps, and government figures suggest that early detection (leading to early treatment) saves over 1,000 lives each year. Women aged under 50 are not routinely invited for screening, partly because breast tissue before the menopause is dense and so mammography is less helpful. It is also the case that breast cancer in women aged under 50 is relatively uncommon: 80% of breast cancers occur in women over 50.

Further information

UK

Cancer Research UK's information on mammograms in breast screening: www.cancerhelp.org.uk/type/breast-cancer/about/screening/mammo grams-in-breast-screening

US

National Cancer Institute information on mammography: www.cancer. gov/cancertopics/factsheet/Detection/mammograms

American Cancer Society: www.cancer.org/Healthy/FindCancerEarly/ ExamandTestDescriptions/MammogramsandOtherBreastImaging Procedures/mammograms-and-other-breast-imaging-procedures-toc

M is for Marie Curie Cancer Care

Established in 1948 – the same year as the National Health Service – Marie Curie Cancer Care is a UK charity dedicated to the care of people with cancer and other terminal illnesses. Its services are always free of charge to patients and their families. There are more than 2,000 Marie Curie Nurses and Healthcare Assistants across the UK, providing end-of-life care for patients at home and support for their families.

The nine Marie Curie Hospices offer specialist care for inpatients. They are in Belfast, Bradford, Edinburgh, Glasgow, Hampstead (London), Liverpool, Newcastle, Penarth (Cardiff) and Solihull. A wide range of outpatient and day services enable the hospices to reach many more local people for whom a hospice bed may not be the best option.

Marie Curie Cancer Care also conducts palliative care research to find better ways of caring for terminally ill people, and the charity campaigns extensively to support patients' decisions to be cared for and die in the place of their choice. This has attracted widespread support from patients, their families and healthcare professionals.

TOP TIP

Marie Curie Cancer Care's website offers film guides which focus on personal care and everyday living for patients and carers. They include practical demonstrations. Visit www. mariecurie.org.uk.

Further information

UK

Contact **Marie Curie Cancer Care** for information about their nursing service. Phone: 0800 634 4520 (free call) seven days a week, 9 a.m. to 10.30 p.m. Marie Curie Cancer Care, 89 Albert Embankment, London SE1 7TP. Website: www.mariecurie.org.uk

M is for Massage

It is easy to dismiss the physiological and psychological benefit of touch, but it is clearly evident in people with cancer. The relaxation of tense muscles, which in turn improves blood and lymphatic circulation and encourages the body to get rid of toxins, can only serve to aid the body's healing processes. The ensuing feeling is one of well-being as anxieties and stress are replaced with reassurance, peace and calm. Another reported benefit is a greater feeling of focus. Regular treatments have shown improved concentration, which is definitely a plus after chemo!

Indian head massage

This technique involves massage of the face and scalp, neck and shoulders. As these areas are known to hold stress and tension, the foremost benefit is relaxation. It's a 'today's world' treatment. For anyone who works at a computer, whose shoulders become raised and stiff from sitting in a certain position for a long time, whose eyes are sore from staring at a computer screen, and who has eyestrain and a throbbing head by the end of the day, such massage is a Godsend. For someone with cancer, there are many more benefits.

Indian head massage was used in India as a beauty treatment, to help women keep their long black hair glossy. Then men found it encouraged thicker, healthier hair growth. If you lose hair during your chemo treatment, this is a great way to encourage beautiful, healthy regrowth. Perhaps more importantly for someone with cancer, Indian head massage can soothe in a way that conventional medicine cannot. It has a personal, hands-on approach (literally) that care based on drugs, technology and efficiency has lost. It is important not to forget the story of the rabbits and how much better they did with a cuddle (see 'P is for Psychoneuroimmunology and the Power of Positive Thought').

Shiatsu massage

Shiatsu massage (*shi* meaning *finger* and *atsu* meaning *pressure*) is a therapeutic technique from Japan with its roots in traditional Chinese massage and Western physical manipulation. Shiatsu is based on the principles of acupuncture but uses pressure from the fingertips, *acupressure*, instead of the insertion of fine needles on the acupoints of the body's meridians. Central to shiatsu is the element of touch through which the practitioner aims to restore harmony between *yin* and *yang*: lack of harmony can deplete or block the flow of *qi* and cause 'dis-ease' (see 'A is for Acupuncture'; 'T is for Traditional Chinese Medicine').

Having made an in-depth assessment of the health and needs of the patient, a practitioner can use a variety of techniques to remove energy blockages. These include gentle holding, pressing with thumbs, fingers, palms of the hands, elbows, knees and feet on the meridians and, if appropriate, more dynamic rotations, stretches and manipulation techniques similar to those practised by Western physiotherapists. Often working on deep tissues, the massage is said to be very relaxing, having a beneficial effect on the whole body and promoting well-being and healing.

In the case of cancer, where advice is generally against deep tissue massage, shiatsu treatment would be of a light, supportive nature with the intention of increasing the overall vitality of the individual by enhancing the flow of bodily energy. The patient generally lies on the floor on a futon and the treatment is applied by touch through loose clothing. By unblocking the stagnant *qi* the practitioner aims to effect physiological improvements to the flow of the lymphatic system and the circulation, release toxins and stimulate the hormone and immune system. After massage it is important to drink plenty of water to help clear the toxins released.

Research and anecdotal evidence has shown that gentle massage can relieve the depression, stress and anxiety associated with cancer and alleviate side effects of chemotherapy treatment regimes such as nausea, fatigue, insomnia and pain. On another level, the release of powerful, long-held emotions, which can occur during or after treatment, may help spiritual healing.

Shiatsu treatments should only be given with the approval of a doctor, by a qualified practitioner, and be seen as a support mechanism not a cure.

Lymphatic drainage massage

Lymphoedema is chronic swelling, usually affecting an arm or leg, which occurs in the case of cancer when a lymph node has become blocked or when part of the lymph system is removed or damaged during surgery or radiotherapy. This impedes the elimination of metabolic waste, toxins and excess fluid from the body by the lymphatic system.

Oedema in the arm frequently follows breast cancer surgery which has involved the removal of lymph nodes or radiotherapy to the armpit. This accumulation of fluid makes it difficult to move the arm and often causes pain and anxiety. Designed to stimulate drainage of excess fluid from the swollen area, treatment includes raising the affected limb, wearing compression garments, special exercises, manual lymphatic drainage (MLD) and skin care.

A specialist lymphatic drainage therapist (see 'Further information') will move the skin in specific directions using gentle and precise hand movements and rhythmic stretching and pumping techniques that relate to the anatomy of the lymphatic system. The aim is to move the excess fluid into an area with working lymph vessels so that it can drain away normally. MLD is often followed by the fitting of compression garments to stop fluid from building up again. Advice will be given on skin care, reducing the risk of infection, and gentle exercises and simple self-massage that can be carried out at home. Increasingly, MLD is provided by the National Health Service at lymphoedema treatment clinics. It is important to contact your doctor or nurse for specialist help at the first sign of swelling.

TOP TIP

Warm sesame oil can be used during a massage but has a strong smell. Coconut oil can be a more pleasing option.

If you have had surgery, avoid wearing tight-fitting clothing, including underwired bras, to encourage lymph fluid to circulate freely.

Further information
UK

General Council for Massage Therapies: 27 Old Gloucester Street, London WC1N 3XX. Tel: 0870 850 4452. Website: www.gcmt.org.uk

Penny Brohn Cancer Care's evidence-based leaflets on *Massage and Shiatsu*, downloadable from www.pennybrohncancercare.org. Follow links from 'Information and Research'.

The **British Lymphology Society** produces a directory of NHS and private lymphoedema centres. 9–11 Oldbury Road, Cheltenham, Gloucestershire GL51 0HH. Tel: 01242 695077. Email: info@thebls.com. Website: www.thebls.com

Manual Lymphatic Drainage UK: PO Box 14491, Glenrothes, Fife KY6 3YE. Tel/Fax: 0844 800 1988. Email: admin@mlduk.org.uk. Website: www.mlduk.org.uk

Macmillan Cancer Support for useful information on lymphoedema. Follow the links from 'Cancer information' to 'Living with and after cancer': www.macmillan.org.uk

Shiatsu Society, PO Box 4580, Rugby, Warwickshire CV21 9EL. Tel: 0845 130 4560. Website: www.shiatsusociety.org

US

American Cancer Society information on massage: www.cancer.org/ Treatment/TreatmentsandSideEffects/ComplementaryandAlternativeMedi cine/ManualHealingandPhysicalTouch/massage, and information on myofascial release: www.cancer.org/Treatment/TreatmentsandSideEffects/ ComplementaryandAlternativeMedicine/ManualHealingandPhysical Touch/myofascial-release

Reference

Medicine Hands: Massage Therapy for People with Cancer by Gayle Macdonald. Findhorn Press (2007).

M is for Mastectomy

Surgical removal of the breast is often recommended when cancer has invaded surrounding tissue or spread to the lymph nodes. This can be followed by reconstruction of the breast, either at the same time as the initial operation, or at some later point. Some women with a strong family history of breast cancer (see 'B is for BRCA1 and BRCA2') choose to have mastectomies to remove all risk that the disease will develop.

A young woman in her 20s telephoned to ask me about mastectomy and reconstruction (see 'R is for Reconstruction of the Breast'). She had such a bad history of breast cancer in her family that she was thinking of having a double mastectomy as a precaution against the disease. It seemed desperately sad that a young woman should have to face such a decision. There are so many possible means of prevention, and of cure, hovering close to the horizon. But she wanted to do everything in her power to avoid a cancer which she had seen kill close members of her family. There is so much – life – at stake.

I was completely horrified when advised to have a mastectomy. The only way I would consider it was with reconstruction. I had limited time to decide, because I was told the operation was urgent. I saw photographs of women 'wearing their mastectomy scar with pride', but I knew this was not me. Many women have a mastectomy with no fuss and no reconstruction. It is a question of knowing yourself – and I knew that I would be emotionally, mentally and physically affected. More importantly, I knew my spirit would be floored. For my survival, I needed to be as positive and upbeat as possible. A reconstruction and the flat tummy from whence the reconstructive tissue came (which would have taken me a lifetime to achieve in the gym) offered the opportunity to turn a negative into a positive. There are pros and cons (discussed under 'R is for Reconstruction of the Breast'). But I was and remain completely adamant that simultaneous reconstruction should be offered to all women as a matter of course.

TOP TIP
I am I and you are you whatever!

Further information
UK

Find out about support groups in your area, advised by your medical care team.

Breast Cancer Care information on breast cancer surgery: www.breastcancercare.org.uk/breast-cancer-breast-health/treatment-side-effects/surgery, and on breast reconstruction: www.breastcancercare.org.uk/breast-cancer-breast-health/treatment-side effects/surgery/reconstruction

US

American Cancer Society information on breast cancer surgery: www.cancer.org/Cancer/BreastCancer/DetailedGuide/breast-cancer-treating-surgery, and information on breast reconstruction: www.cancer.org/Cancer/BreastCancer/MoreInformation/BreastReconstructionAfterMastectomy/index

Reference
Take Charge of your Breast Cancer: A Guide to Getting the Best Possible Treatment by John Link. Henry Holt & Co (2002).

M is for Meditation

Meditation is quite a toughie to describe, let alone to do at first. To meditate is not so much to focus but to de-focus, not so much to concentrate as to allow oneself just to be. It is to let the mind clear, to lose the chattering inner voice and truly relax on all levels. For a cancer patient, whose life is suddenly in turmoil, this place of complete peace – once found – can be like the eye of a tropical storm, a place of respite from the surrounding chaos.

Before my diagnosis, I am not sure I had any real concept of what meditation was. I thought of it as something carried out by people in flowing robes wearing sandals, sitting cross-legged, hands together, sometimes chanting.

I learnt about meditation and how 'to do it' at Penny Brohn Cancer Care (formerly Bristol Cancer Help Centre; see 'P is for Penny Brohn Cancer Care'). At first it was very difficult to switch off the constant chattering of my mind, as ideas, thoughts and plans hurtled through. This is completely normal. One learns that you can simply recognize each thought as a little interruption and then allow your mind's composure to return, without feeling annoyed at yourself. Some people find a mantra (saying the same word or words over and over again) helps. I found it helpful to concentrate on the flame of a candle, thinking of and listening to absolutely nothing except the rhythm of my breathing. Many times I would fall asleep, which was interesting because one of the reasons to meditate as a cancer patient is to bring yourself to your place of calm and peace, optimizing the body's ability to heal itself. Sleeping aids this healing state but is not the prime purpose of meditation.

Nowadays, doctors are increasingly citing stress as a major contributing factor to illness. Research has shown meditation to be beneficial for a wide range of health problems. Reducing stress through meditation, our minds and bodies can begin to function with improved effectiveness.

Meditation is not the same as concentration, or contemplation, and it is not a religion. It is a route – practised for thousands of years – to a far deeper consciousness and awareness, beyond thought. It is a marriage of light, spirituality and guidance. It is not about forcing the mind to be quiet. It is about finding the stillness and silence that is already there.

The practice of meditation shuts out the demands, trivialities, anxieties and concerns of our daily life, allowing us to connect to an inner (much calmer) being and experience a profound sense of our own place within the greater scheme of things. Entering a state of pure awareness, your mind quiets, your body is deeply rested, and learning and healing abound.

How to meditate

There are many forms of meditation and there is no 'best' way. It is thought that half an hour of meditation gives you much more energy than half an hour of sleep. Try not to have any expectations but sit comfortably with your hands in your lap or resting on your thighs, and your eyes closed. Meditate not for the feeling experienced whilst meditating, but for the benefits it can bring to your life for the other 23 hours of the day, for example, to your health, relationships and choices. In Hinduism, it is believed that 'Om' is the primordial sound from which all creation arose and as such is used by many as a silently repeated mantra, but a mantra can just as easily be a meaningless word of your own choice. If you notice your attention drifting, which is perfectly normal, you can gently bring it back to your mantra. As an alternative to sound meditation, you may choose breathing meditation, where you gently place your awareness on the breath entering your body and how that feels, then breathe out. 'So hum' is a breathing mantra. Think 'so' on the in breath and 'hum' on the out breath. You might find it easier, at least initially, to follow a guided meditation, for example, *Soul of Healing Meditations*, a CD by Deepak Chopra.

TOP TIP

The ideal for me is to start and finish the day with a meditation of half an hour. Try this twice a day for three weeks and you will become addicted!

Further information

UK

Penny Brohn Cancer Care evidence-based leaflet on meditation and mindfulness: www.pennybrohncancercare.org/upload/docs/932/medita tion_and_mindfulness.pdf

The School of Meditation, 158 Holland Park Avenue, London W11 4UH. Tel: 020 7603 6116. Email: info@schoolofmeditation.org. Website: www.schoolofmeditation.org

US

Some **Gilda's Clubs** offer free classes in meditation: www.gildasclub. org. The larger cancer treatment centres may include meditation in their Integrative Medicine Programs.

American Cancer Society information on meditation: www.cancer.org/ Treatment/TreatmentsandSideEffects/ComplementaryandAlternative Medicine/MindBodyandSpirit/meditation

References

Breast Cancer Beyond Convention: The World's Foremost Authorities on Complementary and Alternative Medicine Offer Advice on Healing edited by Mary Tagliaferri, Isaac Cohen and Debu Tripathy (particularly chapter 11). Atria (2002).

Being Oneself: The Way of Meditation by F.W. Whiting. The School of Meditation (2001). Order from www.schoolofmeditation.org/beingoneself2.htm.

Soul of Healing Meditations (CD) by Deepak Chopra. Rasa (2004).

Meditation for Beginners (CD included) by Jack Kornfield. Bantam Books (2005).

Teach Yourself to Meditate: Over 20 Simple Exercises for Peace, Health and Clarity of Mind by Eric Harrison. Piatkus Books (1994).

M is for Mind, Body, Spirit and Healing

It could be argued that every illness, disease or accident affects the whole body, mind and spirit. This is true even of a broken arm. It makes the rest of the body work harder to compensate. It limits what you can do and so is dispiriting. And you may wonder whether you will ever have complete use of that arm again, generating feelings of anxiety that can cloud your days.

Of course, the usual approach in the case of a broken arm will be to treat it in isolation. But, with cancer, the problem is much wider. Here, you will always be aware that tumour cells from the primary cancer could be on the rampage, spreading through the blood supply or the lymphatic system to hunt out new homes. In living with cancer, it is important to engage body, mind and spirit in a determined effort to deter them. You *can* do this.

First, the body needs to be given the correct fuel in the form of food to help it function at its best. Your body needs to be looked after and appreciated. And it may need encouragement to use its own resources for healing. It may be that your body has come under stress that has affected the immune system (see 'I is for Immune System and Immunotherapy'). So take things to strengthen immunity if you need them.

Second, every individual has responsibility for their own healing and dealing with their own illness. It is worth taking the time to ask why this illness may have come about, for there may well be reasons. One possibility is that the illness is destined to teach us something: many cancer patients recognize the lessons they have learnt, and some actually regard the experience as a gift of learning. And it may not be teaching the patient alone but also others – the family, carers, even doctors. Another possibility is that the illness is designed to draw attention to some area of your life that has gone wrong, or is not functioning as it should. It may be there to allow opportunities to stop, reassess, and re-evaluate. Perhaps you need to take the time to grieve for someone or something (a death, or divorce, or simply an injustice) in a way that was not possible at the time. Any sort of obsession, whether it be righteous indignation or just a nagging preoccupation diverts the energy of the body from self-healing. So it is important to recognize errors in others as *their* problem, and try not to be too involved in their bad energy.

The body requires plenty of rest and uninterrupted time to plan and to regroup its defences. You may experience fatigue. Don't ignore this important indicator. Is your body crying out for some peace and quiet so that it can get on with healing? Often when the 'fatigue' bell goes for me, I get under my duvet and say to my body, 'OK. Now you have time for the body's own intelligence to go to work.' And I try to stay in a 'mindless' state, in the knowledge that what I am thinking influences my body on a cellular level – particularly if I am worrying about something stressful.

The mind, therefore, must be stilled for healing. Sleep is good. Steady breathing can help (see 'B is for Breath and Breathing'). Or use the mind to your advantage, to help the body rid itself of cancer (see 'V is for Visualization'). Agree between your mind and body what you are trying to do and why. If all else fails and you are lying there unable to stop panicking, BE FIRM. Breathe – and try and imagine a wonderful white light coming straight from the heavens to zap your cancer. To help, I try and position myself to capture a sun beam, beamed on an appropriately chosen spot – either to recharge, or to zap!

Healing of the spirit is perhaps the most important and the most neglected of all aspects of healing. Spirit cannot be allowed just to cooperate. You need to be *enthusiastic* about your survival and getting shot of this cancer, and about your good health and well-being. This usually means you have to be enthusiastic about Life (see 'L is for Life'). A spirit that is bored, defeated and feeling a victim of the disease is making life more difficult. There are several reasons why your spirit's heart may not be in this recovery. Are you lonely in your everyday life, or depressed, or feeling – as we all do from time to time – deflated and of little or no worth? Once you have recognized the problem or problems, whether it be an overstressed immune system due to lifestyle, or a fed-up spirit due to life, you can do something about it (see 'C is for Control'). This may even be the time to consider spiritual healers.

It is important for the spirit to be having fun, so you need to spend time doing the things you love – whether it's being in your potting shed or painting. And you do not have to do this on your own: most spirits like company, so think of how you can do things with others.

TOP TIP

It is quite an ordeal keeping on top of all your medical appointments and treatments. You need your home team – mind, body and spirit – on your side. You may identify with what I have written and see the areas where you need help. If not, do seek some help – it's there for you. Also, some enlightened National Health Service Trusts do employ spiritual healers.

Further information

UK

Penny Brohn Cancer Care evidence-based information sheet on healing: www.pennybrohncancercare.org/upload/docs/932/healing.pdf

Confederation of Healing Organisations (CHO) Tel: 01584 890662 Website: www.confederation-of-healing-organisations.org

The National Federation of Spiritual Healers, now known as **NFSH The Healing Trust**, 21 York Road, Northampton NN1 5QG. Tel: 01604 603247. Website: www.thehealingtrust.org.uk

Cancer Research UK: www.cancerhelp.org.uk/about-cancer/treatment/complementary-alternative/therapies/healing

Cancer Recovery Foundation UK: www.cancerrecovery.org.uk

References

The Healer's Manual: A Beginner's Guide to Energy Therapies by Ted Andrews. Llewellyn (2005); especially Chapter 2, 'The Occult Significance of the Body'.

Born to Heal: Guidance and Insight from an Extraordinary Irish Healer by Tony Hogan. Random House (2002).

You Can Heal Your Life by Louise L Hay. Hay House UK (2004).

Anything can be Healed by Martin Brofman. Findhorn (2003).

Cancer as a Turning Point: A Handbook for People with Cancer, Their Families, and Health Professionals by Lawrence LeShan. Gateway (1992).

Treating Body, Mind and Soul: Alternative Solutions for Modern Living by Jan de Vries. Mainstream (2003).

Nine Ways to Body Wisdom: Blending Natural Therapies to Nourish the Body, Emotions and Soul by Jennifer Harper. Thorsons (2000).

The Endorphin Effect: A Breakthrough Strategy for Holistic Health and Spiritual Wellbeing by William Bloom. Piatkus (2001; new edition expected November 2011).

The Healing Journey: Overcoming the Crisis of Cancer by Alastair J. Cunningham. Healing Journey Books (2010).

Why Do People Get Ill? Exploring the Mind–Body Connection by Darian Leader and David Corfield. Penguin (2008).

Spiritual Healing and the Appliance of Science by B.H. Smith, Department of General Practice and Primary Care, University of Aberdeen, Foresterhill Health Centre, Westburn Road, Aberdeen AB25 2AY. Tel: 01224 553972. Email: blairsmith@abdn.ac.uk.

M is for Mistletoe

You may have thought it's just for kissing under, but this seasonal plant has had a long history of association with magic and healing. In the 1920s, Rudolf Steiner proposed mistletoe as a treatment for cancer as part of the anthroposophical approach to medicine. This system, which developed from homeopathy, was based on the idea that disease is caused by imbalance in the body and that treatment should restore natural healing. Part of the attraction of using mistletoe may have been the analogy between its status as a parasite of plants and cancer as a parasite in people.

Mistletoe has an interesting chemistry and contains substances that may inhibit tumours and stimulate the immune system. However, this highly toxic herb is not suitable for self-medication.

Mistletoe extracts can kill cancer cells in the laboratory and have been shown to affect the immune system. But it is difficult to confirm the efficacy of mistletoe against real tumours, though there have been studies in animals and some trials in patients (see the Cancer Cure Foundation website www.cancure.org/iscador_mistletoe.htm for more information). Mistletoe products are widely used in Germany to treat cancer, and a group of doctors from Nuremberg recently assessed all the evidence they could find from controlled trials. Their conclusion, published in the *Cochrane Database Systematic Review* in 2008, was that there is some evidence mistletoe extracts can improve quality of life, reduce symptoms and help with the adverse effects of chemotherapy. The evidence such treatment can extend survival in patients with cancer was regarded as weak. The German authors encouraged people wanting to take mistletoe products to participate in further clinical trials. But such trials seem few and far between.

Cancer Research UK says that the mistletoe product Iscador can boost white cells, but that 'there is no study evidence it can slow or cure cancer'.

Further information

UK

NHS Evidence – Complementary and alternative medicine: www.library.nhs.uk/cam/SearchResults.aspx?searchText=mistletoe&tabID=289

Anthroposophic Health, Education and Social Care Movement, c/o Camphill Medical Practice, Murtle Estate, Bieldside, Aberdeen AB15 9EP. Tel: 01224 869621. Website: www.ahasc.org.uk

Weleda UK, Heanor Road, Ilkeston, Derbyshire DE7 8DR. Tel: 0115 944 8222 for supplies and a list of prescribing doctors. Email: sales@weleda.co.uk. Website: www.weleda.co.uk

The integrated care service of the **Royal London Hospital for Integrated Medicine** offers a range of complementary therapies, including the prescription of oral or injectable mistletoe preparations, on the National Health Service. Website: www.uclh.nhs.uk/OurServices/ServiceA-Z/INTMED/IMCAN/Pages/Home.aspx

US

Lewis Gale Hospital website. Scroll down to 'Natural and Alternative Treatments' on the main menu and click on 'Herbs and Supplements'. Then find 'Mistletoe' in the A–Z list: www.alleghanyregional.com/healthcontent.asp?page=contentselection/condensedmainindex

Memorial Sloan-Kettering Cancer Center: www.mskcc.org/mskcc/html/69305.cfm

EU

Lukas Clinic, Arlesheim, Switzerland. Tel: +41(0)61 702 09 09. Website: www.lukasklinik.ch

Reference

Iscador: Mistletoe in Cancer Therapy by Christine Murphy. Lantern Books, US (2001).

M is for Monoclonal Antibodies

When a white blood cell (or lymphocyte) recognizes a 'foreign' protein (or antigen) on the surface of invading bacteria or viruses, or on one of our own cells that is abnormal, it produces an antibody. This is a highly specific response: a single lymphocyte produces one antibody, and that antibody alone.

Thirty years ago, scientists in Cambridge (UK) found that they could fuse a single lymphocyte with a cell from a bone cancer. The resulting hybrid cell combined the ability of a normal lymphocyte to produce a specific antibody with the cancer's capacity for survival, allowing a cell line to be grown in the lab. Because the line derives from a single parent cell, which makes identical copies (clones) of itself, the antibody it produces is called monoclonal.

High on the list of priorities was the production of monoclonal antibodies that could home in on molecules present on the surface of specific cancer cells. An antibody tagged with a radioactive tracer and injected into a patient will concentrate at sites where the cancer is present, and this technique is proving valuable in detecting tumour spread. It is also enabling doctors to direct radiation and anti-cancer drugs specifically at cancer cells, leaving their healthy counterparts undamaged. Such targeted therapies are used in several forms of blood and marrow cancers (see 'L is for Leukaemia' and 'L is for Lymphoma').

Monoclonal antibody drugs (their names end in the suffix 'ab', for antibody) have also proved helpful in treating breast cancer (trastuzumab, or Herceptin, being the prime example), and cancer of the colon (where cetuximab, or Erbitux; and bevacizumab, or Avastin) are used.

Further information
UK

Cancer Research UK: www.cancerhelp.org.uk/about-cancer/treatment/biological/types/about-monoclonal-antibodies

US

Monoclonal antibody information from the **Mayo Clinic**: www.mayoclinic.com/health/monoclonal-antibody/CA00082

N is for Naturopathy

Whilst the term was first used in the UK and US in the nineteenth century, much of the philosophy behind naturopathy is in the teaching of Hippocrates (460–375 BC). Central to this is the idea that the body can heal itself naturally if given the opportunity to do so, and that the cause of disease is the body being out of balance. The way to keep it in balance was (and is) to eat simple natural food and take regular exercise. In the twenty-first century, the basic tenet of using the healing power of nature still stands, but naturopathy incorporates our growing wealth of knowledge about health and the human body. As a holistic (see 'H is for Holistic') approach, naturopath physicians treat the whole person (mind, body and spirit) using herbs, nutrition and homeopathy. They also pay attention to lifestyle and psychological issues.

The holistic approach may mean conducting certain diagnostic tests that do not seem related to the patient's specific complaint. One example might be a blood test which can detect exposure to pesticides. The physician will be seeking to assess the state and condition of the whole body by its reaction.

Much naturopathic medicine centres on the liver. This is because when the liver cannot function properly, toxins – instead of being eliminated from the body – recirculate and cause further damage. Bearing in mind the strain imposed on the liver by toxins introduced into the system to kill cancer, making a priority of supporting liver function may well be extremely useful.

Further information
UK

British Naturopathic Association, 1 Green Lane Avenue, Street, Somerset BA16 0QS. Tel: 01458 840072. Email: admin@naturopaths.org.uk. Website: www.naturopaths.org.uk. The Association has a specialist oncology group.

US

National Center for Complementary and Alternative Medicine: http://nccam.nih.gov/health/naturopathy

American Association of Naturopathic Physicians (please note although the term physician is used, it does not mean the person has attended a traditional medical school): http://naturopathic.org

A sceptical view on naturopathy from **Quackwatch**: www.quackwatch.org/01QuackeryRelatedTopics/Naturopathy/naturopathy.html

References

What Really Works in Natural Health by Susan Clark. Bantam (2004).

Nine Ways to Body Wisdom: Blending Natural Therapies to Nourish the Body, Emotions and Soul by Jennifer Harper. Thorsons (2000).

N is for Nausea

Nausea and vomiting (or, in medical terms, 'emesis') are natural responses when our bodies are exposed to toxic substances. Both anti-cancer drugs and radiation are highly toxic, and both can damage the rapidly dividing cells that make up the lining of the stomach. But the idea that everyone is nauseous with chemotherapy is simply myth. Cancer is a very individual disease, and the effects of the drugs are also individually felt. Also, some chemotherapy drugs and combinations are more likely to induce nausea than others (cisplatin and paclitaxel being particularly likely to have this side effect).

If you do experience nausea, then the first point of call is the oncologist. The days of being a quiet, long-suffering patient are gone. There are many different ways that chemotherapy drugs can be given, and there is a huge range of anti-nausea drugs. One or other of them is going to suit you.

Many patients these days are given an anti-emetic drug that works by inhibiting a nausea centre in the brain that is activated by serotonin. Examples are Kytril (granisetron) and Zofran (ondansetron). The 2009 annual meeting of the American Society of Clinical Oncology heard the results of a trial demonstrating that patients taking ginger capsules along with these anti-nausea drugs had fewer symptoms than those taking a dummy placebo pill. The effective dose was equivalent to a quarter to half a teaspoon of ground ginger. Where all else has failed, acupuncture also has success in preventing nausea and vomiting (see 'A is for Acupuncture').

I have had various cocktails of chemotherapy and have never felt nauseous. This may be because of the anti-nausea drugs. It could be because I was careful to be as relaxed as possible when taking the chemotherapy. It could be because I am an expert on sea sickness and have found that it is a good idea to have something in your stomach – be it dry biscuit or sweet biscuit. If sickness is experienced in the morning, be ready with a tin of biscuits by the bed. Having something fruity (such as fruit pastilles) helps, and I have heard that this is also true of rinsing the mouth with carbonated or fizzy water. Ginger is a natural antidote to nausea and I find it helps to eat crystallized ginger or dunk ginger biscuits in a cup of tea. Ginger ale also settles queasiness very well. Foods to avoid include anything greasy, fried or hot and spicy: sometimes the smell of it can be enough. I noticed that the Penny Brohn Cancer Care (formerly Bristol Cancer Help Centre) sells 'Sea-Bands' – wristbands with an acupressure point which helps in the prevention of nausea.

Further information
UK
Penny Brohn Cancer Care Tel: 01275 370 112. Website: www.shop atpennybrohn.com

US
Information on nausea and vomiting from the **National Cancer Institute**: www.cancer.gov/cancertopics/pdq/supportivecare/nausea/Patient

N is for Neoadjuvant Therapy

Sometimes chemotherapy (or hormone therapy in the case of breast cancer) is given before an operation. Termed neoadjuvant therapy, this is usually done in an attempt to reduce the size of large tumours so that surgery becomes possible, or so that less of the healthy tissue has to be removed. For example, neoadjuvant chemotherapy has been used successfully to shrink breast tumours and allow lumpectomy rather than mastectomy. It is also used in some patients with prostate cancer. Neoadjuvant therapy in throat cancer may allow the voice to be preserved, and it can enable certain patients with cancer of the rectum to avoid the need for a permanent colostomy.

Neoadjuvant treatment also has the advantage of establishing whether a particular tumour is responsive to chemotherapy. This can be comforting if chemo is going to be used after surgery to mop up any escaped cancer cells which are running around looking for a new home. The disadvantage is that you have to steel yourself while waiting for definitive surgery in the knowledge the chemo may not work and the cancer might be spreading. Neoadjuvant therapy is also pretty intensive and time-consuming and can have significant side effects.

Further information
UK
Cancer Research UK: www.cancerhelp.org.uk/about-cancer/cancer-ques tions/what-is-down-staging

N is for Neuro-Linguistic Programming (NLP)

Neuro-Linguistic Programming, co-founded and promoted in the 1970s by Americans Richard Bandler and John Grinder, is a powerful form of brief psychotherapy that taps into the subconscious and enables transformation to take place. It is a useful tool in changing repetitive and sometimes destructive behaviour and thought patterns. It is commonly used to make behavioural changes relating to overeating, binging on chocolate, phobias, emotional problems, pain management and chronic fatigue.

It can also help change behaviours and thought patterns that are extremely unhelpful for someone with cancer, such as panic attacks, depression and stress. The idea is to replace negative, destructive responses with a more empowered, forward-looking way of being.

Anyone with cancer can have a treatment protocol tailored to suit his or her unique requirements. This is then continually evaluated. So, throughout the cancer journey, NLP is a continued source of support, dealing with crisis points as they occur – from initial diagnosis, through treatment, to improved health and living with cancer.

TOP TIP
This is terrific and life-changing.

Further information
UK

Linda Crawford: linda@allergyline.com

NLP World: www.nlpworld.co.uk/anlp-abnlp-inlpta-and-other-affiliation-bodies

The Professional Guild of NLP, a non-profit making and non-commercial organisation, seeks to provide an interface between quality NLP training and the public at large. Tel: 0845 226 7334. Website: www.professionalguildofnlp.com

The **Association for Neuro-Linguistic Programming (ANLP)** seeks to offer an independent service to NLP professionals and the general public: www.anlp.org

US

See co-founder **Richard Bandler's** website: www.nlplifetraining.com

References
Making a Difference in Cancer Care: Practical Techniques in Palliative and Curative Treatment by Claire Rushton. Souvenir Press (1994).

'Applications of neurolinguistic programming to medicine' by J.F. Christensen and colleagues. *Journal of General Internal Medicine* 1990, volume 5, pages 522–527.

N is for NICE

The National Institute for Health and Clinical Excellence (NICE) is an independent body, but funded by the UK government. Founded in 1999, its role is to decide which drugs the National Health Service (NHS) can afford, based on efficacy, which – in the case of cancer drugs – is often measured as cost per life-year gained. The idea was that it should establish norms that prevented regional disparities in the availability of expensive new drugs – the so-called 'postcode lottery'. But its decisions apply to England, and not to Scotland and Wales. So geographical disparities have continued.

There were great hopes for this organization when approval of the breast cancer dug Herceptin (trastuzumab) was fast-tracked. In August 2006, this new antibody drug was approved as a way of reducing the risk of disease recurrence in women with a particular kind of breast cancer (HER2-positive). But NICE proved reluctant to allow Velcade (bortezomib) to be used in patients with the bone marrow cancer multiple myeloma, and did not approve Avastin (bevacizumab) for bowel cancer. The controversy has continued with the new kidney cancer drug Sutent (sunitinib), which was not allowed to be used by the NHS until a year or more after it had been approved in most of the rest of Europe. The integrity of NICE, particularly its freedom from government influence, has been called into question.

It is argued that the amount of money available for healthcare is finite, which is true, but there is room for debate about the proportion of the government's budget assigned to the NHS and about the overall level of taxation. Many people also feel betrayed that, having dutifully paid into the health system, too little money is available for their treatment once the need arises. These problems are particularly acute with a life-threatening condition like cancer and when new but very expensive drugs are continually becoming available. It is hard for a patient to accept that a treatment costs too much for the NHS to afford.

A
B
C
D
E
F
G
H
I
J
K
L
M
N
O
P
Q
R
S
T
U
V
W
X
Y
Z

N is for Noni Juice

Noni juice is derived from the fruit of the tropical tree *Morinda citrifolia* and has been widely used as a traditional medicine. Stories of the health-giving benefits of the noni fruit are plentiful in French Polynesia, for example. Its important constituents seem to be plant sterols such as sitosterol. Studies have suggested that men consuming a low-fat, high-fibre diet containing high amounts of plant products have a lower risk of prostate cancer than those who do not, and laboratory work has shown some anti-cancer effect in mice. Anti-inflammatory and anti-thrombotic effects have also been claimed.

I was diagnosed with a serious liver problem. On a liver function test, the level of one important enzyme (ALT, alanine transaminase) was 800. (Normal values would be somewhere between 5 and 50.) Two biopsies were performed and I was told that I should need steroids for the rest of my life. The side effects looked horrendous so I decided to look for an alternative in the form of milk thistle and noni juice. Some three years later, the ALT count was down to 42. I took the juice under the watchful eye of my own doctor and continued to be monitored in case of a relapse.

Further information

UK

Organic Noni Juice available from **Natural Juices**: www.naturaljuices.co.uk

US

For a sceptical view from **World Wide Warning** of the pyramid selling and celebrity endorsement that underlie some noni juice sales, see: http://noni.worldwidewarning.net/index.php

Reference

The Noni Solution: The Juice Millions of People Drink to Achieve Optimal Health and Wellness by Neil Soloman. Direct Source Publishing (2004).

N is for Nutritional Therapy

See 'D is for Diet and Nutritional Therapy (or Food, Glorious Food)'

P is for Peace

> May the peace of God, which passeth all understanding, be with you.

So we say, most of us, without any clear understanding of what we are saying.

In my pre-cancer days, I might have thought we were talking about world peace, peace amongst nations. But now I know what I mean when I use those words. I mean an inner peace with which I am so content and safe – in the knowledge that whatever happens, everything (in my world and for me) is going to be OK. In fact, more than OK. When you have experienced THAT peace, even for a fleeting moment, it is much treasured, not least because you know it is there. Some say it is a connection with the universe and deep understanding of one's place in the scheme of things.

To bring about such peace, you need to have calmed your spirit. The constant inner chatter needs to be muted. Some people find this inner state through meditation (see 'M is for Meditation') and some through prayer.

In my case, I have first to silence my thoughts and empty my mind of all daily trivia (and things that are not so trivial) so that I am floating in a peaceful state. To help, I concentrate on my breathing (see 'B is for Breath and Breathing'), and then Peace cometh like dew on a new born leaf.

Further information
Reference
Pure Bliss: The Art of Living in Soft Time by Gill Edwards. Piatkus Books (2006).

P is for Penny Brohn Cancer Care

Penny Brohn was diagnosed with breast cancer in 1979. She recognized the isolation, fear and uncertainty that such a diagnosis brings and saw the need for an integrated, holistic approach that would support people living with cancer, their loved ones and carers. Developed along with her friend Pat Pilkington, the result was the Bristol Cancer Help Centre offering 'the Bristol Approach'. Now known as Penny Brohn Cancer Care, the charity offers specialist support including complementary therapy, nutritional advice and counselling. There is a wide range of residential courses available for people living with cancer and their carers or supporters. There are also courses for health practitioners.

In February 2003, my prognosis with inflammatory breast cancer was grim, and I decided to attend a one-week course at the Bristol Centre. I found it invaluable in so many ways.

To start with, I was systematically and methodically assessed not only for diet but also for my state of mind. Reading the claims that diet cannot cure or control cancer, yet knowing how much better I feel on the Bristol diet, I am convinced that we are in a much better position to win through when we have a diet that puts little or no stress on the system or body.

It makes sense to avoid foods containing chemicals and concentrate on wholefoods, fresh foods and vegetables – organic where possible. The exception might be a glass – or two – of wine. Sadly, this was banned during the week's course, but I have to admit feeling so much better without my usual intake of alcohol and caffeine, which is the other banned substance.

I was nervous about attending the group therapy sessions, and I think everyone felt the same apprehension to start with. But in no time I found great strength from being part of such a special group of people and made some very solid friendships. It was as if the experience of cancer was binding us together in a unique way.

I also attended individual sessions with a psychotherapist, a homeopathic doctor, a Reiki or spiritual healer and had various sessions of reflexology and aromatherapy.

When the time came to leave, I am not sure that I realized the transformation that had taken place in me whilst in the care of these professionals. The panic or near panic I had felt and the feelings of isolation, of going through this on my own were completely gone. They had been replaced with a sense of peace and that 'all is well' with the world, and an understanding of a greater scheme of things. Looking back, it was an integral part of a rather late spiritual awakening. And, of course, I had been detoxed and felt physically great.

TOP TIP
Turn to Penny Brohn Cancer Care – *now*!

Further information
UK
Penny Brohn Cancer Care, Chapel Pill Lane, Bristol BS20 0HH. Freephone: 0845 123 23 10, 9.30 a.m. to 5 p.m. weekdays. Website: www. pennybrohncancercare.org

Reference
Anti-cancer: A New Way of Life by David Servan-Schreiber. Michael Joseph (2008).

P is for Personality

It *seems* only common sense that a fighting spirit should affect the outcome of cancer, as of many aspects of life. But it has proved surprisingly difficult to demonstrate by research. There is evidence that a coping style which is characterized by helplessness and lack of hope is associated with an unfavourable outcome in certain cancers. But evidence for the converse – that a fighting spirit leads to a better outcome – is less clear-cut. At least, these were the findings of a study at the Royal Marsden Hospital which measured psychological response to the diagnosis of breast cancer in almost 600 women and followed them for many years. Women with a helpless/hopeless response initially were less likely than others to be alive after five or ten years. Women whose early response was categorized as 'fighting spirit' were no more likely than others to do well. (But see also 'P is for Psychoneuroimmunology and the Power of Positive Thought' for evidence that guided imagery can enhance the immune response.)

Further information
References
'Influence of psychological response on breast cancer survival' by M. Watson and colleagues. *European Journal of Cancer* 2005, volume 41, pages 1710–1714.

'The Tyranny of Positive Thinking' by Jimmie Holland: www.humansideofcancer. com/chapter2/chapter.2.htm.

P is for Pesticides

See also 'C is for Chemicals'

Pesticides are designed to kill pests and diseases that eat and damage crops – and our food. The idea is that, by spraying, the farmer can guarantee more yield per acre of more perfect crops, and the consumer can buy more perfect goods at an economic price because there is little wastage (i.e. no pitmarked or bug-marked items).

Are pesticides actually essential or cost-effective? Let's take the case of the perfect English apple. Using pesticides, there will be no sign of a disastrous attack of blight, of woolly aphid, red spider mite or codling moth. And, somewhere between picking and arrival on the supermarket shelf, it may also have been dipped in waxy 'polish' which not only extends its shelf life in the supermarkets, but makes the apple appear rosy, shiny and totally irresistible. But isn't the reality that lacewings absolutely adore woolly aphids, and parasitic wasps equally adore red spider mite, and codling moth can be deterred by tying a wide band of sticky tape around the lower trunk of the tree? And is it not also the case that by the time you have paid for the pesticide or insecticide, hired the equipment or serviced and maintained the sprayer, hired the labour or spent the time yourself spraying (and, of course, this is at the convenience of the weather – which must not be too wet because the sprayer tractor gets stuck in the mud, or be before a downpour because the spray dilutes and ends up in the ground, and must not be too windy because there is spray 'drift' and it ends up everywhere except on your trees), the costs may not be so different?

But maybe this is a digression. The real issue is whether pesticides can cause cancer. A link has been found by Dr Charles Charlier, a toxicologist at Sart Tilman Hospital in Liège, Belgium. In 2003 he reported that blood levels of dichlorodiphenyltrichloroethane (DDT) were significantly higher in women with breast cancer than in women without the disease. DDT has been banned in England but its effects can continue for some 50 years. Pesticides have also been linked to Parkinson's disease, ME, multiple sclerosis, epilepsy and Alzheimer's – with cases being reported from residents close to the spraying activity. Particularly vulnerable are unborn children, developing children and the elderly. The Royal Commission suggested a five-yard buffer zone but the Government's advisory committee on pesticides apparently did not recommend its implementation.

The evidence about the health damage caused by organophosphates generally centres on neurological problems. The jury is out on whether there is any clear link between other forms of pesticides and cancer. The people most at risk are probably those who mix and apply the pesticides, or the children of farm workers. But Cancer Research UK say that the evidence for higher rates of cancer in agricultural workers is inconclusive, and the enhanced risk – if any – would be small.

In one study, researchers from the California Department of Health took data for every square mile in the state and tested to see if there was a relationship between incidence of cancer and density of pesticide use. They concluded there is little evidence of higher cancer rates among children with greater exposure to pesticides. However, a more recent study from the US shows that people exposed through their work to certain pesticides have twice the usual risk of developing an abnormality of certain white blood cells which may be a precursor of multiple myeloma, an uncommon blood marrow cancer.

With regard to self-reported household use of pesticides, there are several reports suggesting links with leukaemia and brain tumours, but bias is difficult to exclude from such studies.

TOP TIP

If it's a windy day and you see a farmer spraying in the distance – get out of there! Be safe: buy organic or grow your own.

Further information
UK

Royal Commission on Environmental Pollution (RCEP), Room 108, 55 Whitehall, London SW1A 2EY. Tel: 0300 068 6474. Email: enquiries@ rcep.org.uk. Website: www.rcep.org.uk

Pesticide Safety Directorate (PSD) Tel: 01904 455775. Email: pesticides@hse.gsi.gov.uk. Website: www.pesticides.gov.uk

Advisory Committee on Pesticides (ACP) Tel: 01904 455702. Email: acp@hse.gsi.gov.uk. Website: www.pesticides.gov.uk/acp.asp

The Soil Association, South Plaza, Marlborough Street, Bristol BS1 3NX. Tel: 0117 314 5000. Website: www.soilassociation.org

US

National Cancer Institute information on pesticides: http://progressreport. cancer.gov/doc_detail.asp?pid=1&did=2007&chid=71&coid=713&mid

P is for Photodynamic Therapy

Photodynamic therapy starts with administration of a light-sensitive but at this stage inactive agent. This becomes concentrated in cancer cells since they are more metabolically active than normal ones, although the agent is present in the whole body. A specific wavelength of laser light is then used to activate the photosensitive drug and the tumour is destroyed with little damage to surrounding normal tissue. The photosensitive agent can be given into a vein or, in the case of skin cancer, applied as a cream. Where the cancer is in a body cavity such as the oesophagus or stomach, the laser light can be directed onto it using a fibreoptic tube, or endoscope. In the prostate, hollow transparent tubes are placed into the prostate through the skin and laser fibres placed into the tubes.

Unlike radiation, there is no limit to how much photodynamic therapy you can have. It does not involve surgery or hospitalization and can be used repeatedly. In its early development, the main drawback was that the photosensitizing agents remained in the body for several months, requiring you to stay out of sunlight. Now, they are usually eliminated after about 24 hours and sensitivity to sunlight is only an issue for a few days. Photodynamic treatment has been licensed for head and neck cancers for five years and is under evaluation for prostate cancer.

Cytoluminescent therapy differs from standard photodynamic therapy in its choice of sensitizers. Instead of using the 'first generation' drug photofrin, it uses green plant-based sensitizers. These are said to be more effective and less toxic.

TOP TIP

This is a good example of a treatment where the side effects may be alleviated by the integration of a complementary approach. Ask a medicinal herbalist about astragalus (see 'A is for Astralagus').

Further information
UK

National Medical Laser Centre (NMLC) at University College London, 1st Floor, Charles Bell House, 67–73 Riding House Street, London W1W 7EJ. Tel: 020 7679 9060. Email: med.laser@ucl.ac.uk. Website: www.ucl. ac.uk/surgicalscience/departments_research/gsrg/nmlc

US

National Cancer Institute, 'Photodynamic therapy for cancer – questions and answers': www.cancer.gov/cancertopics/factsheet/Therapy/photodynamic

References

'Photodynamic therapy: A clinical reality in the treatment of cancer' by C. Hopper. *Lancet Oncology* 2000, 1212–9.

'The application of photodynamic therapy in the head and neck' by W. Jerjes and colleagues. *Dental Update*, October 2007.

Battling Cancer – with Light! by Lev G. Fedyniak MD, 24 November 2003: www. cancerlynx.com/cancerlight.html.

P is for Pilates

Physical fitness is the first requisite of happiness. In order to achieve happiness, it is imperative to gain mastery of your body. If at 30 you are stiff and out of shape, you are old. If at 60 you are supple and strong, then you are young.

Joseph Pilates (1880–1967)

The Pilates Method, or 'Contrology' as it was first known, was designed by Pilates to improve overall core stability and posture. The six underlying principles are breathing, centering, concentration, control, precision and flowing movement. Inspired by the classical Greek ideal of a man who is balanced in body, mind and spirit, it is this holistic approach that sets Pilates apart. It is also widely considered safe and sensible for all ages and fitness levels.

German-born Pilates' interest in health stemmed from his determination to overcome his own problems. Frail and sickly as a child, he became a competent martial artist, gymnast, diver and skier. He devised a unique sequence of movements designed to work the mind and body in harmony – targeting the deep postural muscles to rebalance the body and bring it into alignment. The body is thereby allowed to function more efficiently, building strength, flexibility, stamina and coordination. Later, while interned on the Isle of Man during the First World War and working as a hospital orderly, he turned his attention to rehabilitating bed-ridden patients and created a series of light resistance exercises by rigging springs on hospital beds – the inspiration for his famous equipment, the 'Reformer'.

In 1920s New York, his method became popular with dance legends aiming to improve their technique and/or recover from injury while developing long, lean and elegant muscle. The Pilates Method continues to be endorsed by celebrities including Darcey Bussell, Kate Winslet and Daniel Craig and is now widely available at health clubs.

In 1945, Pilates wrote *Return to Life Through Contrology* outlining his 'intelligent exercise' method where the mind is used to 'control' the body. Today, the Pilates Method is widely respected by the medical profession for the treatment of a range of conditions including back pain, sports injuries, incontinence, osteoporosis, arthritis, multiple sclerosis and stress-related illnesses. Teachers of Pilates often work closely with GPs, osteopaths and physiotherapists (it is not unusual for physiotherapy practices to have an in-house studio where Pilates is taught).

As the Pilates Method can be modified to accommodate any injury, imbalance or weakness, it can help patients to regain their physical confidence after a diagnosis of cancer, surgery or chemotherapy, rebuild their self-esteem and start on the road to recovery. Active involvement in one's own well-being can combat the loss of control often associated with cancer. Concentration and breathing techniques can also help with pain management and treatment of side effects (see also 'B is for Breath and Breathing').

For breast cancer patients, Pilates exercises can be adapted to help restore mobility to the shoulder area following surgery. Lymphoedema or swelling in the arm – caused by fluid build-up associated with the removal of lymph glands in breast surgery – can also be relieved (see 'Lymphatic drainage massage' under 'M is for Massage'). Repeated muscle contractions promote lymph node drainage while diaphragmatic breathing techniques relax the body as a whole, balance stress levels, remove waste from cells and reoxygenate the blood.

TOP TIP

The emphasis should be on the quality not quantity of exercise!

As with any exercise programme, it is important to check its suitability with your doctor and to find a comprehensively trained teacher (see 'Further information' below).

Further information
UK

The Australian Physiotherapy and Pilates Institute (APPI), Lower Ground Floor, 50–52 Kilburn High Road, London NW6 4HJ. Tel: 020 7372 3606. Website: www.ausphysio.com. For teachers of modified Pilates who are also trained physiotherapists.

Body Control Pilates, 35 Little Russell Street London WC1A 2HH. Tel: 020 7636 8900. Fax: 020 7636 8898. Email: info@bodycontrol.co.uk. Website: www.bodycontrol.co.uk. For instructors trained to Level 3 Pilates with current membership of the UK Register of Exercise Professionals. Also Pilates equipment.

A
B
C
D
E
F
G
H
I
J
K
L
M

Pilates Foundation, Administrator, PO Box 58235, London N1 5UY. Tel: 020 7033 0078. Email: admin@pilatesfoundation.com. Website: www. pilatesfoundation.com

US

Cancer patients are urged to avoid inactivity and guidelines for exercise were published in 2010. Information from the **National Cancer Institute** can be found at: www.cancer.gov/ncicancerbulletin/062910/page5

United States Pilates Association: www.unitedstatespilatesassociation. com

References

Pilates for Breast Cancer Rehab (DVD). Stott Pilates (2008).

Pilates Body Control (DVD) by Lynne Robinson. Firefly Entertainment (2009).

The Mari Winsor Pilates for Pink Workout (DVD). Gaiam (2008).

Pilates' Return to Life Through Contrology by Joseph H. Pilates. Presentation Dynamics, illustrated edition (1998).

The Complete Classic Pilates Method: Centre Yourself with This Step-by-step Approach to Joseph Pilates' Original Matwork Programme by Miranda Bass, Lynne Robinson and Gordon Thomson. Pan Books (2005).

P is for Placebo

N
O
P
Q
R
S
T
U
V
W
X
Y
Z

When trying to assess the benefits and risks of a new drug, doctors are aware that patients' expectations can have an important effect on outcome. So their studies contain a comparison group which is given something that looks just like the drug but contains inactive ingredients. This 'dummy' pill is called a placebo (the word is Latin for 'I will please'). For the clinical trial to be free of bias, it is important that neither the patient nor the doctors assessing the results know which patients have had the real drug and which the placebo (see 'C is for Clinical Trial').

Being given something you expect to work sometimes makes it work (or makes it work at least a bit). At times, people think of this 'placebo effect' in a negative light: gullible patients have been fooled into something. But it is not like that at all. There is nothing negative in patients' faith that doctors will help them, and nothing negative in doctors accepting that what a patient thinks or believes can make a difference to the outcome. In fact, it is very positive: doctors are acknowledging that you may be able to influence the course of your disease and help recovery. As the Roman philosopher Seneca (4 BC–AD 65) put it: 'It is part of the cure to wish to be cured.'

The placebo effect is most clearly seen with treatments that are aimed at reducing or preventing pain, and it is widely thought that the body's own opiate-like chemicals (endorphins) are involved. That said, we do not really understand what is happening at a cellular level when someone's belief that they have been given an active drug actually achieves at least part of the aim of treatment.

In clinical trials for cancer, patients in the control group (against which the new treatment is compared) generally receive not a placebo but the best treatment currently available (often called the 'standard of care'). Only in that way is it possible to tell with reasonable certainty whether or not the new treatment marks a genuine advance.

I can quote an extremely good example of how belief in a doctor can help. I went to see a professor at the Royal Brompton Hospital about the possibility that my cancer had spread to the lung. Breathing was difficult and I was quite down about it. He said he did not recommend any intervention. My body was coping well with the fluid in the lung, which was most likely a short-term consequence of surgery, but we'd keep an eye on it. I came out a changed woman. The cause was probably not metastatic spread. I felt fine, and from then on my breathing was amazingly improved. We had instantly established a good therapeutic relationship and I totally believed what he said.

Further information
Reference

The Human Effect in Medicine by Michael Dixon and Kieran Sweeney. Radcliffe Medical Press (2000).

A
B
C
D
E
F
G
H
I
J
K
L
M
N
O
P
Q
R
S
T
U
V
W
X
Y
Z

P is for Polarity Therapy

Polarity involves opposites, as in 'poles apart'. Polarity therapy is a form of manipulating energy. It acknowledges that we are surrounded by a huge force-field and are ourselves made up of energetic matter. There is polarity interwoven with the very fabric of our lives – hot/cold, positive/negative. But between the poles of these dimensions is a middle state: warmth in one case, neutral in the other. Polarity therapy negotiates this middle ground in order to optimize health: energy moves from a positive to a negative pole through a neutral field.

It was developed 60 years ago by Dr Randolph Stone, an osteopath, chiropractor and naturopath. He felt that symptoms were a result of blockages, much as when a river stopped from flowing causes a pool of stagnant water. True healing can take place only if the free flow of energy is restored. This is also the philosophy of both Ayurvedic and Traditional Chinese Medicine. The polarity healer seeks to find the 'blockage' through bodywork, emotional and mental support, polarity yoga, and health-building and cleansing diets.

Our own energy is affected by all aspects of our lives – physical, mental, emotional and spiritual – and good health depends on all these areas being in harmony. So polarity therapy also aims to bring these energies into a state of balance. It incorporates and relies on many healing traditions from East and West, ancient and modern, to form an integrated and effective healing art.

Further information

UK

UK Polarity Therapy Association, Monomark House, 27 Old Gloucester Street, London WC1N 3XX. Website: www.ukpta.org.uk/polarity. Visit this website to find a polarity therapist near you.

US

American Polarity Therapy Association: www.polaritytherapy.org

References

'Polarity Therapy: Linking Ancient Knowledge and Modern Physics' by Will Wilson, June 2000. Website: www.positivehealth.com/articles/polarity-therapy/230.

Polarity Therapy: Healing with Life Energy by Alan Siegel and Phil Young. MasterWorks International (2006).

The Polarity Process: Energy as a Healing Art by Franklyn Sills. North Atlantic Books (2002).

P is for Power and Patient Power

A hospital can be the perfect place to practise the misuse of power. If a patient is late, make 'em pay, make 'em wait. If a patient decides she is a better judge of what is good for her than an 18-year-old rather bossy nurse – woe betide. 'Madam, the nurse has blacklisted you with her colleagues, and they consider you a challenge. They are doing everything in their power to make your life difficult – to break you. So obey.' OK, that scenario is the exception. It stands out against the general background of compassion and care. But it sometimes happens. Power freaks can be attracted to being in charge of the most vulnerable in our society: the elderly and, of course, the sick. The other compassionate and caring staff may fear the obvious confrontation and lack the strength of character to stand up to these few.

Then you listen to certain senior people making decisions about which drugs the National Health Service is going to allow (spend money on), and you realize that this is yet another opportunity for abuse of power. You expect the doctor to be the one responsible for deciding which drugs you need and trust that the doctor has no other agenda. But this is not always so. As someone with cancer, as a carer or as a professional in the field of cancer, you need to be aware of these issues and have the courage to stand up for what you believe to be right.

Let me cite a personal example. When I'd already encroached by about six months on the two years it was supposed that I would live, I attended a certain chemotherapy outpatient unit where one or two of the 'senior' (aged about 18) nurses apparently saw me as a 'challenge' and were attempting to bring about change – for my spirit 'to be broken' so that I would sit quietly and malleably whilst they kept me waiting from

8.30 a.m. until 4.00 p.m. for my two hours of then weekly chemotherapy treatment. When the acting senior nursing officer for the hospital arrived to tell me this, I was totally in despair – I could not believe that anyone facing a major life-threatening disease could be so badly let down by two or three singularly immature young nurses, seemingly left to their own devices (or vices) to run the chemo department of a major London hospital with a very fine reputation for cancer care. It seemed that the nursing officer was not intending to hold these nurses responsible in any way, or to rebuke them for their evil behaviour towards me. The weak creature bleated something about how hard it was to find staff... It was a totally depressing experience and the effect on me was that I was extremely depressed.

The dilemma was how to continue with my brilliant oncologist, yet not to have the actual treatment at that hospital. My oncologist was the key and he made the arrangements for treatment at an alternative hospital. Now the treatments are every three weeks and I look forward to going because I know I am amongst friends whom I can literally trust with my life. The moral: if there is a problem of this kind, change the faulty component of the team. No one needs negative or unhelpful 'attitude' problems. Everyone deserves the perfect patient/cancer carer relationship (whether it is with a professor or the most junior nursing assistant), not least because that very relationship MAY well have an impact on your well-being and even chances of survival.

TOP TIP

A significant aspect of power is your own power. If you are in a vulnerable state as a patient, it is difficult to imagine you have any power at all – but you do! Don't put up with shoddy or unsympathetic treatment.

Further information

UK

Macmillan Cancer Support, 'Making a complaint': www.macmillan. org.uk/Cancerinformation/Cancertreatment/Gettingtreatment/Making acomplaint.aspx

P is for Prayer

As a Christian, I derive immense support from prayer, and not only the prayers I say myself. Luckily for me (and I did not know this until my own diagnosis of cancer), I am surrounded by many extremely devout pray-ers. Thankfully, I have featured in their prayers. What is this power of prayer, and how can it help?

I see it as a hugely positive force (see 'E is for Energy'). I also feel the energy of group consciousness, of collective prayer or chanting – so much the greater when it takes place in a church or other sacred site (see 'References' below: *The Field*, pages 267–269).

Scientific evidence that the power of prayer aids healing is somewhat lacking. The review 'The healing power of prayer and its implications for nursing' (*British Journal of Nursing*, March 2008) concludes in its abstract that 'although the evidence for the healing power of spirituality is inconclusive, there are indications that it has potential for the health and wellbeing of both patients and nurses'.

Further information
References
The Field: The Quest for the Secret Force of the Universe by Lynne McTaggart. Element (2003).

The Link Between Religion and Health: Psychoneuroimmunology and the Faith Factor by Harold G. Koenig. Oxford University Press (2002).

P is for Presents

Just in case anyone wants to know the best presents to give someone with cancer, I suggest these (all in the pampering category):

• slippers which have a microwavable insert and are cream
• the fluffiest, hugest bath towel

- the fluffiest towel robe after a bath or shower
- a favourite aromatherapy oil if known – or a sample set to try
- a naturally scented candle
- a fun hot water bottle
- a pashmina or shawl to throw around your shoulders in bed
- *Experience Yoga Nidra* (CD) – a deep guided meditation by Swami Janakananda.

Further information

UK

Dr Lisa Maddison, founder of **Get Well Gifts**: www.getwellgifts.co.uk/department/gifts_for_cancer_patients

Penny Brohn Cancer Care: www.shopatpennybrohn.com

US

A number of companies selling gifts specifically for cancer patients can be found online. Two examples are **CancerGifts.com**: www.cancergifts.com, and **The Pampered Patient**: www.thepamperedpatient.com

P is for Prostate Cancer

The prostate is a small gland (about the size of a walnut) that sits like a collar around the urethra, the tube that carries urine from the bladder to the penis. Its secretions contribute to the seminal fluid on ejaculation. Most men experience some enlargement of the prostate as they age, and this can make it difficult to urinate. But difficulty in urination, reduced urine flow and the need to pass water frequently during the night could be symptoms of prostate cancer and need to be checked out by a doctor. On the other hand, many men with prostate cancer have no symptoms at all, which makes it difficult to detect without screening (discussed in detail below).

Each year, over 36,000 men in the UK are diagnosed with prostate cancer – a number fast catching up with the 45,000 women diagnosed with breast cancer – which makes it the most common cancer in men by a clear margin. In the US, there are now almost 220,000 cases of prostate cancer each year, which is more than the number of newly diagnosed breast cancers. Prostate cancer in a man's father or brother increases the chances that he will develop the disease.

Diagnosis and treatment

Two tests suggest the possibility of cancer. The first is a high level in the blood of a substance produced by prostate cells called prostate-specific antigen (PSA). The second is when a doctor can feel a lump or irregularity in the prostate by inserting a finger in the rectum (a procedure known as digital rectal examination). But the disease can only be diagnosed with certainty by a biopsy: a fine needle is used to take tissue samples from the prostate, and the tissue is then examined by microscope in a pathology lab. If there is a prostate cancer, doctors will use the way the cells appear under the microscope to assign a 'Gleason score' to the tumour. This provides some evidence of how likely the cancer is to spread and is one of the factors used to suggest the best treatment.

If the tumour is small and confined to the prostate and has a low Gleason score, doctors may suggest simply that they keep a careful check on it with repeat PSA tests and rectal examination. When a tumour is likely to become a problem if left untreated, the main options are either radiotherapy (using an external beam or radioactive seeds implanted in the gland – see 'B is for Brachytherapy') or surgery. Where the cancer has not spread outside the prostate, there is now some evidence that cryosurgery (in which probes destroy malignant tissue through extremely low temperature) is as effective as external beam radiation (see 'C is for Cryotherapy').

If the cancer has spread into tissues around the prostate itself or to other parts of the body (it is quite common for prostate tumours to set up secondary cancers in the bones, for example), the mainstay of treatment is hormonal therapy. This is designed to counter the effects of testosterone, which makes prostate cancers grow. Hormone therapy has two main forms. One is the use of monthly or three-monthly injections of an LHRH agonist such as Zoladex or Prostap. These drugs are 90–95% effective in preventing the body producing testosterone. A second form of hormone therapy is use of daily anti-androgen tablets which block the effects of testosterone on the prostate cell. The two kinds of drug can be used together and with radiotherapy. Hormonal treatment has potential side effects such as hot flushes, erectile dysfunction and enlargement of the breasts. But it usually keeps prostate cancer under control, at least for a while.

If prostate cancer progresses despite hormone therapy, chemotherapy may help. But there are many side effects. So there is great interest in the first convincing evidence of benefit from a different and much less toxic form of treatment. In 2009, we heard the first results of a large American trial of an activated cell vaccine (see 'I is for Immune System and Immunotherapy'). In this study, 500 men whose advanced prostate cancer no longer responded to hormones were assigned to two groups. Both had a specific form of immune system cell extracted from their blood. The job of these 'dendritic' cells is to become aware of substances (antigens) on a cell showing that it is foreign (like a bacterium) or malignant and bring this to the attention of the immune system's attack troops. Patients in the active vaccination arm had their dendritic cells exposed to an antigen found on most prostate cancer cells before being reinfused. Patients in the placebo arm received their cells back without them being primed with antigen.

On average, men who had the active vaccine (called Provenge) lived four months longer than those who did not. Active cellular immunotherapy also resulted in a 38% improvement in the chances of being alive after three years: in the Provenge-treated group, 32% of men were alive, compared with 23% in the control group. Because it is tailored to the individual patient, such vaccination is expensive. It may be that it is too expensive to be used widely outside certain very specialized centres in the United States, where Provenge has been approved for use. But the results of this trial are regarded as highly promising for patients with advanced prostate cancer and for those with other tumours – because it proves in principle that we can harness our own immune systems in the fight against the disease.

There is also great interest in a new drug called Abiraterone which stops the body producing testosterone. The results of a large trial in men with advanced prostate cancer have been very encouraging and many specialists believe that Abiraterone will greatly improve patients' prospects.

Why prostate screening is not straightforward

A big question – much debated by doctors but still unresolved – is whether it would be a good idea to screen men for prostate cancer. Unlike mammography to detect possible breast tumours, prostate screening would not involve an X-ray. Instead, there is a simple blood test to measure the level of prostate-specific antigen (PSA).

Over 15 years ago, a major study in the United States started the mammoth task of assigning almost 80,000 men (aged between 55 and 75) at random either to a screening group who were offered annual measurements of PSA or to a control group who were not. After a decade, the death rate from prostate cancer in the screened group was no lower than that among men who were not offered regular PSA checks. That is perhaps a disappointing outcome. But the good news is that the death rate from prostate cancer (about two deaths per 10,000 man-years) is low among both groups of men. A possible reason for the failure to show that a screening programme makes a difference is that about 40% of the men who were not invited each year for a PSA test chose to have one anyway, and so also enjoyed the benefits of being tested.

That is probably part of the explanation. One reason for thinking so is the result of a similar study carried out over the same period in Europe, where men were much less likely to have organized their own PSA testing. An even larger number of men (160,000) were randomized to either PSA screening (once every four years on average) or no screening. In this study, the death rate from prostate cancer among men given screening was 20% lower than among those who did not have PSA tests. This difference was statistically significant, which is to say it was very likely a true effect of screening and not one that arose by chance. But the benefit in absolute numbers was small: to prevent one man dying from prostate cancer, you would have to screen 1,400.

Well, why not screen 1,400? The answer is that screening also has some disadvantages (in addition to its cost). Among the 1,400 men screened, there would be 49 in whom prostate cancer was detected. All would experience the profound anxiety caused by such a diagnosis. The majority would have some form of treatment, and some men would undergo months (if not years) of living with the consequences of surgery, radiotherapy and drugs. The bottom line is that 48 men would experience adverse effects without any benefit in order that one has his life saved.

Some doctors think that PSA screening should be offered to all middle-aged men. Some think it should be restricted to men judged to be at above-average risk. Others argue that testing is largely a waste of time until we are able to distinguish reliably between small prostate cancers that are going to grow aggressively – and so pose a threat to life – and those that are not. Much effort is being spent on identifying the molecular and genetic features that demonstrate a prostate tumour is one that is going to spread. But we are not there yet.

Further information
UK

Cancer Research UK Freephone: 0808 800 4040 to speak to a cancer information nurse. Website: www.cancerhelp.org.uk/type/prostate-cancer

Macmillan Cancer Support: www.macmillan.org.uk/Cancerinformation/ Cancertypes/Prostate/Prostatecancer.aspx

Prostate UK, 6 Crescent Stables, 139 Upper Richmond Road, London SW15 2TN. Tel: 020 8788 7720. Email: info@prostateuk.org. Website: www.prostateuk.org

US

PSA Rising: www.psa-rising.com

National Cancer Institute: www.cancer.gov/cancertopics/types/prostate

Prostate Cancer Foundation: www.pcf.org

Prostate Conditions Education Council: www.prostateconditions.org

Prostate Cancer Research Institute: www.prostate-cancer.org/pcricms

Us TOO International Prostate Cancer Education and Support Network: http://ustoo.org

References

The Far End of Fate: A Humorous Diary of the Symptoms, Diagnosis, Treatment and Side Effects of My Prostate Cancer by Graham A. Newman. Prostate Research Campaign UK (2006).

The Prostate: Small Gland, Big Problem, a booklet available from Prostate UK (see above).

'A randomized trial of external beam radiotherapy versus cryoablation in patients with localized prostate cancer' by B.J. Donnelly and colleagues. *Cancer* 2010, volume 116, pages 323–330.

P is for Psychoneuroimmunology and the Power of Positive Thought

This newish 'ology' made its debut around 1981. The basic premise is that the body has a biochemical or physical response to every thought we have. Just think of how shutting your eyes and imagining a fearful situation can change your pattern of breathing and make you sweat, and contrast that with the effects of imagining yourself on a deserted beach listening to the gentle breaking of the waves.

As far as living with cancer is concerned, the hope is that positive thought will result in a better biochemical response than negative thought and that it can be used to support the immune system. Stress can change the way the immune system responds and may well have an influence on survival. Natural killer cell and T cells are part of the body's immune response to cancer and a randomized controlled trial has now shown that relaxation and guided imagery increase the number and activation of such cells to a statistically significant extent.

But you feel how you feel, and there is little point in pretending to be optimistic because this is said to boost your immune system, or in feeling in any way guilty because you're desperately depressed by the diagnosis, prognosis or even the ongoing cancer treatment. There are lots of helpful tools in the tool box: choose the one best suited to your own task.

That said, it is much easier to be a positive person if you are surrounded by positive people. Weed out your negative friends and ban them from your presence! And if those whom you prop up don't get the message that it's now your turn for support, banish them too. You know who they are: they start the conversation with 'How are you?', but two seconds later you are discussing *their* problems. Although you may love them, this is the time when you must conserve your energy and think of yourself.

It is becoming more usual for a psychologist to be a part of the cancer care team, so that when patients feel overwhelmed and depressed by their diagnosis or prognosis, there is help at hand in the form of psychological therapy. But help does not have to take the form of sophisticated intervention.

There is a lovely story. Two sets of rabbits were being used for research and no one could understand why one set of rabbits was coping with treatment so much better than the other set – until one researcher was caught giving the 'better' set of rabbits their daily cuddle while the other researcher simply plonked her batch back in their cages.

When waiting for my own diagnosis, I cleaned and reorganized every cupboard in the house, incessantly telling my husband where everything was. In a way, this was extremely positive – we had a house full of clean cupboards. On the other hand, it was negative – since I obviously thought I would not be around to find things for him.

On the day I was diagnosed, I read in the paper that an estate agent had been shot showing an applicant around a property in Belgravia, London. His life was over. Mine was not. And I realized that actually I felt quite lucky.

Positive thoughts and emotions such as love and laughter are to be encouraged, while negative thoughts such as fear and disappointment are to be discouraged. You can create positive thoughts by spending time with people you love and who love you. You can also seek out the things that make you laugh. Fear and disappointment are much trickier and, like the cancer itself, less controllable. With a diagnosis of cancer, the first thoughts are usually along the lines of, 'It's such a shame because I won't be able to do X and Y.' Rather perversely, I found an empowerment: 'As I have a rather bad prognosis, I am absolutely going to do X and Y. And I absolutely will not be wasting time doing Z.' This caused a few upheavals in our household.

TOP TIPS

Walk into the light – literally. If you have any dark thoughts, go into the sunlight if you can, or at least turn the light on. Imagine being bathed in a white healing light. Practise this so you can use it whenever you have negative thoughts.

Further information

References

'Psychoneuroimmunology: A new fad or the fifth cancer treatment modality?' by Leslie Walker and Oleg Eremin, *The American Journal of Surgery* 1995, volume 170.

'Immuno-modulatory effects of relaxation training and guided imagery in women with locally advanced breast cancer undergoing multimodality therapy: A randomized controlled trial' by O. Eremin and colleagues, *Breast* 2009, volume 18, pages 17–25.

For an essay arguing that people sometimes go overboard in thinking that a fighting attitude and positive outlook will affect outcome, see 'The Tyranny of Positive Thinking' by Jimmie Holland at www.humansideofcancer.com/chapter2/chapter.2.htm.

The Biology of Belief: Unleashing the Power of Consciousness, Matter and Miracles by Bruce Lipton. Hay House (2008).

Q is for Qigong

Qigong (see also 'T is for Tai Chi') is one of China's oldest forms of therapy. It dates back over 5,000 years to the days of the Yellow Emperor and is strongly linked with Traditional Chinese Medicine. Inspired by the instinctive, flowing movements of wild animals, the ancient Qigong exercises are integral to the philosophy of following the way of harmony with nature and least resistance, and were historically practised by Taoist and Buddhist monks to aid concentration and martial arts training. Qigong consists of two Chinese words, *qi* and *gong*. *Qi* is translated as 'breath' but more importantly as 'universal life force' connecting human beings with nature; and *gong* means the time, effort and discipline acquiring a skill.

In Chinese medicine, disease, or 'dis-ease', is believed to develop in areas of stagnation, deficiency or disharmony of *qi* in the body. The practice of Qigong combines sequences of slow, graceful movements to stretch the muscles, tendons and ligaments, with controlled deep breathing, meditation and visualization to stimulate and balance the flow and distribution of *qi*. The underlying principle is to maintain a posture with the minimum of muscle tension, which in itself constricts the flow of energy through our body. Qigong is thought to increase vitality and promote self-healing by bringing blood, oxygen and vital energy to every part of the body. Considered a holistic, mind–body therapy working on a subtle, energetic level, Qigong may also induce a calmer, more harmonious attitude to life.

A more static form of exercise than Tai Chi, Qigong, essentially meditation in motion, can be performed with very little movement at all – standing, sitting or lying down. This makes it especially beneficial for patients suffering from circulatory or respiratory illness, ME, multiple sclerosis, chronic fatigue or cancer. Qigong's emphasis on slow movement accompanied by long, deep breathing and conscious relaxation activates the parasympathetic nervous system and promotes its 'rest and renewal' functions. It is thought to reduce stress and improve the health of the immune system, nervous system and internal organs.

Qigong is no stranger to controversy. Passed down in secrecy by monks, physicians and teachers for many generations, the practice was outlawed during Mao Tse Tung's Cultural Revolution (1966–1974). As recently as 1999, all large Qigong gatherings, viewed as a threat to political and religious stability, were banned by the Chinese government. Today, however, China is anxious to preserve and promote the valuable aspects of its traditional medicine, and Qigong is considered an important therapeutic technique. Traditional Chinese hospitals generally have a Qigong department where masters harness their own *qi* to aid patients' recovery through strengthening massage, whilst teaching patients to work with their own energy to improve their health.

Amongst studies indicating benefits such as decreased heart rate, blood pressure and circulating stress hormones, and enhanced immune function, a recent controlled trial of medical Qigong in cancer patients indicates that the practice improves quality of life, fatigue and mood, and reduces nausea, sleep disturbance and inflammation (see 'Further information' below). Additional studies examining the long-term benefits of medical Qigong, including a potential impact on survival, may provide additional information to assist patients and clinicians in optimizing comprehensive cancer care. The popularity of Qigong in the field of complementary medicine is growing throughout the Western world, as is respect for its efficacy.

TOP TIP

The emphasis is on the quality not quantity of exercise! Focus on your breathing. Once this is working for you, everything will begin to fall into place.

Further information
UK
Tai Chi Finder, 21 The Avenue, London E11 2EE. Tel: 020 8819 2767. Website: www.taichifinder.co.uk

UK Taiji Qigong Foundation: www.uktqf.co.uk

London Academy of Qigong and TCM Tel: 020 8748 1456. Fax: 020 8741 6345. Email: Tcmqigongacademy@yahoo.co.uk

Qi Gong (**Devon School of Tai Chi** DVD) by Matthew Rochford; buy from www.taichifinder.co.uk

To view the graceful **Wild Goose Qigong (Dayan)** Parts 1 and 2 performed by Master Lu Gui Rong: www.youtube.com/watch?v=Jk8yOpqYpgI, and www.youtube.com/watch?v=g5bjpsxdUXY

US

Qigong Association of America: www.qi.org

National Qigong Association: http://nqa.org

Some of the larger cancer treatment centres offer Qigong as part of their integrative medicine programmes. Free Qigong classes may be available at local cancer support programmes such as **Gilda's Club**: www.gildasclub.org

References

The Theory and Practice of Taiji Qigong by Chris Jarmey. Lotus Publishing (2003).

Chinese Medical Qigong by Tianjun Liu and Kevin W. Chen. Singing Dragon (2010).

Managing Stress with Qigong by Gordon Faulkner. Singing Dragon (2010).

Managing Depression with Qigong by Frances Gaik. Singing Dragon (2009).

'Impact of Medical Qigong on quality of life, fatigue, mood and inflammation in cancer patients: A randomized controlled trial' by B. Oh and colleagues. *Annals of Oncology* 2010, volume 21, pages 608–614, http://annonc.oxfordjournals.org/content/21/3/608.abstract.

Q is for Quantum Healing

Quantum, in the context of healing, is a form of 'inner knowing how to heal'. We all have this but have been conditioned not to trust or believe in it because we only 'know' what can be scientifically proved. Deepak Chopra MD, an expert in this field, has experienced 'spontaneous' cures of cancer. In his book *Quantum Healing* (see 'References' on the following page; page 15), he writes:

Research…has shown that just before the cure appears, almost every patient experiences a dramatic shift in awareness. He knows that he will be healed, and he feels that the force responsible is inside himself but not limited to him – it extends beyond his personal boundaries throughout all of nature... At that moment, such patients apparently jump to a new level of consciousness that prohibits the existence of cancer. Then the cancer cells either disappear, literally overnight in some cases, or at the very least stabilize without damaging the body any further.

This idea of connectedness is found in many other philosophies of healing – energy healing, for example. Even meditation encourages you to try and become as one with your surroundings, 'rooted' in Mother Earth, whilst allowing your inner consciousness to connect to a higher source. The quantum leap is one of belief. If you believe and trust that the body can heal itself, can it happen? It does if you break a leg. But we know all too well that cancer can kill, which causes major doubt that the mind can control this disease.

TOP TIP

When I was a child and really hated a certain subject at school, I would do an Oscar-winning performance of someone with a headache, usually resulting in having a headache. We all accept the existence of psychosomatic disease, so what is the problem in accepting that the body has the power to heal itself, even of cancer?

Further information
References

Ask and it is Given: Learning to Manifest Your Desires by Esther and Jerry Hicks. Hay House (2005, reprinted 2008).

Quantum Healing: Exploring the Frontiers of Mind/Body Medicine by Deepak Chopra. Bantam (1990).

Body Intelligence: Creating a New Environment by Ged Sumner. Singing Dragon (2009).

The Biology of Belief: Unleashing the Power of Consciousness, Matter and Miracles by Bruce Lipton. Hay House (2008).

A
B
C
D
E
F
G
H
I
J
K
L
M
N
O
P
Q
R
S
T
U
V
W
X
Y
Z

R is for Radiotherapy

Radiation is the spreading out of energy, just as ripples spread out when a stone is thrown in a pond. Sound, light, radio and TV signals are all examples of radiation. As with the ripples, all radiation has a wavelength – the distance from the top of one wave to the top of the next. Radio and TV signals are the long wavelength end of the radiation spectrum. Visible light is somewhere in the middle. And the radiation used to treat cancer (X-rays and gamma rays) is at the short wavelength end. Unlike visible light, short wavelength radiation can penetrate tissue, and this is most obvious when X-rays are used to reveal a broken bone. Exposure to X-rays used in diagnosis has to be very carefully controlled because this form of radiation also damages tissue. It can, for example, cause the strands of DNA to break. Putting this destructive power to controlled use is the essence of radiotherapy.

Radiation damages all tissues. But it has the greatest effect on cells that are dividing rapidly, as in cancers. Chemotherapy also targets rapidly dividing cells (see 'C is for Chemotherapy'), but radiation has the advantage that it can be directed very precisely so that it hits the tumour while having little effect on the rest of the body. The corresponding disadvantage is that it treats only one site of disease: if the cancer has spread widely through the body, then it has to be treated with drugs.

Surgery, radiation and drugs are the three main pillars of conventional cancer treatment. They each have strengths and weaknesses, and, of course, they are very often used in combination. A clear example is in breast cancer. If the tumour is small, it can be removed with a little surrounding tissue, leaving most of the breast intact. But the operation has to be followed by a course of radiotherapy to mop up any small clumps of cancer cells that may cause the tumour to recur in the breast. And there may also be a need for drug treatment to reduce the chances of new tumours being formed by cancer cells that have spread to other parts of the body.

In other circumstances, radiotherapy is an *alternative* to surgery. Certain prostate cancers can be just as effectively managed with radiotherapy as with surgery, and with less risk of complications such as incontinence and impotence. And some tumours occur in parts of the body which are difficult to operate on, in which case radiation can be invaluable.

Radiotherapy can be given by inserting a radioactive source into the tumour, or placing one close to it. This is done in the case of some prostate cancers, for example (see 'B is for Brachytherapy'). The rest of this section describes *external* radiotherapy. In this form of treatment, the radiation source is in a machine some distance from the patient, and the radiation is directed at the body in the form of a beam. The total amount of radiation to be given is precisely calculated by a radiation oncologist to achieve maximum effectiveness against the tumour while minimizing risk of side effects. The total dose is generally divided into daily amounts (a process called fractionation) and given over a period of several weeks. The precise treatment plan is tailored to the needs of the individual patient. Establishing exactly where the tumour is through various forms of scanning is a key part of the process.

During a planning appointment prior to therapy, the area of the body to be targeted by the radiation beam is mapped: tiny dot marks – tattoos in fact, but almost invisible – are made on the skin. The 'map' and beams can then be lined up very quickly for each treatment. Typically, the radiotherapy machine will rotate around your body, so that beams come in from different angles. The radiation dose is highest at the point where the beams intersect at the site of the tumour. The simulation session also determines how radiation-sensitive areas of the body can best be protected using blocks. This simulation appointment is slightly tedious for the patient because you have to lie very still whilst the calculations and mapping take place, but it is essential that this groundwork is carried out to perfection. You can rest content in the knowledge that once perfectly set up, the actual treatment, which takes place on a daily basis, is incredibly quick and efficient.

The side effect most complained of is fatigue (see 'F is for Fatigue'). If radiotherapy is applied to the head, hair loss can result as the radiation cannot distinguish between the fast-growing cells of the tumour and those of the hair follicle (see 'W is for Wigs'). Reddening and soreness of the skin can also occur. All of these side effects are generally short-term and they are unlikely to be severe.

I had 21 radiotherapy sessions, together with hyperthermia (see 'H is for Hyperthermia') once or twice a week, and am pleased to report few or no side effects. Most radiotherapy departments run an efficient appointment system and I found sessions first thing in the morning the best for me. After half an hour, I had the rest of the day in front of me. You could arrange for sessions to be on the way home from something, or on the way to a film in the early evening. Wherever possible, I have tried to avoid a cancer treatment being the focus of the day.

Improved ways of delivering radiotherapy are opening up new applications. A site of cancer spread that is particularly difficult to deal with is the brain. This organ is very sensitive to radiation damage, and the amount of treatment that can be given using whole-brain radiotherapy is very limited. So there is always interest in new devices that increase the accuracy with which we can deliver treatment. Two such devices – called the Cyberknife and the Gamma Knife, to convey the precision with which they are used – look promising as ways of treating cancers in the brain that have spread from tumours in other organs, as well as in dealing with cancers that have begun in the brain and returned after surgery.

TOP TIP

My absolutely top tip to prevent reddening of the skin is huge applications of aloe vera skin gel (see 'A is for Aloe Vera'). The key to any cancer treatment is to stay well and feel well throughout the treatment, paying particular attention to diet and supplements such as are suggested in Chris Woollams' book (see 'References' on the following page).

Further information

UK

Macmillan Cancer Support: www.macmillan.org.uk/Cancerinformation/Cancertreatment/Treatmenttypes/Radiotherapy/Radiotherapy.aspx

For information from **The Royal Marsden** about radiotherapy treatment and side effects: www.royalmarsden.nhs.uk/cancer-information/treatment/radiotherapy

US

National Cancer Institute information on the following:

Radiation therapy: www.cancer.gov/cancertopics/factsheet/Therapy/radiation

Support for people with cancer: www.cancer.gov/cancertopics/coping/radiation-therapy-and-you

Radiation therapy side effects: www.cancer.gov/cancertopics/coping/radiation-side-effects

American Cancer Society information on radiation therapy: www.cancer.org/Treatment/TreatmentsandSideEffects/TreatmentTypes/Radiation/RadiationTherapyPrinciples/index

References

The Chemotherapy and Radiation Therapy Survival Guide: Information, Suggestions and Support to Help You Get Through Treatment by Judith McKay, Nancee Hirano and Myles E. Lampenfeld. New Harbinger Publications (1998).

Everything You Need to Know to Help You Beat Cancer by Chris Woollams. Health Issues (2005).

R is for Reconstruction (of the Breast)

Removal of the breast (see 'M is for Mastectomy') is an accepted, indeed necessary, way of treating some cancers. For most women, though, the decision to go ahead with it is a dreadful one, and mastectomy should only be offered together with reconstruction. The choice for the patient should be whether to have reconstruction of the breast at the same time as the mastectomy or after all other treatment (such as radiotherapy) has been completed. Reconstruction can also be helpful when only part of the breast has been removed.

The breast can be reconstructed either by using a silicone implant or by taking fatty tissue and muscle from another part of the body. This tissue can be literally flapped over – so tissue from the fatty part of your back forms the new breast (latissimus dorsi flap). The same applies to a flap from the stomach (referred to as a TRAM – transverse rectus abdominis muscle – flap). Flaps can also be taken from the buttock (superior or inferior gluteal artery perforator flaps). These flaps remain attached and the tissue is swung round or channelled into place.

There is also a 'free flap' method where tissue from the abdomen is completely removed together with its own blood supply and then used almost as a patch (DIEP – deep inferior epigastric perforators – flap). This technique is still highly specialized and requires microsurgery skills to reconnect the blood vessels, so it is not universally available.

Immediate and deferred reconstruction both have pros and cons. For me, it was essential that I awoke after my mastectomy with my reconstruction already in place. The bonus was a lovely flat stomach as the tissue had been taken from there. The drawback of immediate reconstruction is that any radiotherapy may make the new tissue slightly lumpy. And that brings worry about the nature of the lumps – is it more cancer? Biopsy gives a fairly definitive answer, but sticking needles into the reconstructed breast can cause tissue to die, resulting in a wound that does not heal well.

Further information
UK
Breast Cancer Care UK: www.breastcancercare.org.uk/breast-cancer-breast-health/treatment-side-effects/surgery/reconstruction

Macmillan Cancer Support: www.macmillan.org.uk/Cancerinformation/Cancertreatment/Treatmenttypes/Surgery/Breastreconstruction/Breast reconstruction.aspx

Macmillan also publish a booklet, *Understanding Breast Reconstruction.*

US

American Cancer Society information on breast reconstruction: www.cancer.
org/Cancer/BreastCancer/MoreInformation/BreastReconstructionAfter
Mastectomy/index

Breastcancer.org: www.breastcancer.org/treatment/surgery/reconstruction/
types

Reference

Take Charge of your Breast Cancer: A Guide to Getting the Best Possible Treatment by John
Link. Henry Holt (2002).

R is for Reflexology (or Reflex Zone Therapy)

The term is used both for a relaxing therapeutic foot massage
and for a curing, restoring method for treating disease.

The theory is as follows: every zone of our body is replicated
as a zone on the foot, predominantly on the soles of the feet.
The condition of the body zones is mirrored in the foot zones, so
that a heavy night's partying, for example, results in a sore liver
zone on the foot. This sensitivity is caused as toxins crystallize
in the relevant foot zone. Gentle massage disperses them to the
lymph system which feeds into the blood and then they are
eliminated from the body by the kidneys. So reflexology aids
in cleansing and restoring balance, which has implications for
the immune system. Reflexology is regarded by some as 'fine
tuning' to promote optimum health and peak performance.

*My first experience of reflexology was in my 20s, when childhood asthma
and hayfever returned with a vengeance. I had deliberately failed to
mention this to my therapist. As he pummelled his way around the bottom
of my foot, I was beginning to think reflexology a complete waste of time.
But then he reached the zone responding to asthma and I almost hit the
roof with the sudden pain. To which he responded, 'A little asthmatic, are
we?' He continued to treat me once a week for a couple of months. I had
no more asthma and considerably improved hayfever for about 20 years.*

Reflexology is clearly a useful diagnostic tool, though not necessarily to be used in isolation. It also worked for me as a cure for asthma.

For those of us living with cancer, there seems to be a general reluctance on the part of therapists to use reflexology in any other way than as gentle foot massage. This certainly gives a feeling of well-being. But it falls well short of what I believe is possible using this approach.

TOP TIP

Be clear about what you require. Is it a gentle foot massage to help with anxiety and create a sense of well-being before, during or after your chemotherapy? Or do you want your therapist to fully address any imbalances or telltale signs of trouble in your body?

Further information

UK

See the evidence-based National Clinical Guideline for the NHS in Scotland for the control of pain in adults with cancer from the **Scottish Intercollegiate Guidelines Network**: www.sign.ac.uk/guidelines/full text/106/index.html

Penny Brohn Cancer Care evidence-based information sheet on Reflexology: www.pennybrohncancercare.org/upload/docs/932/reflexology.pdf

British Reflexology Association, Monks Orchard, Whitbourne, Worcester WR6 5RB. Tel: 01886 821207. Email: bra@britreflex.co.uk. Website: www.britreflex.co.uk

The Association of Reflexologists, 5 Fore Street, Taunton, Somerset TA1 1HX. Tel: 01823 351010. Email: info@aor.org.uk. Website: www.aor.org.uk

US

Reflexology Association of America: www.reflexology-usa.org

For a critical look at reflexology see **Quackwatch**: www.quackwatch. org/01QuackeryRelatedTopics/reflex.html, and **The Skeptic's Dictionary**: www.skepdic.com/reflex.html

R is for Reiki

Reiki (pronounced ray-key) is Japanese for 'universal life energy': *rei* is spirit or spiritually guided, and *ki* is subtle energy. This energy flows around and through all living things and is harnessed through the Reiki master as an entirely safe, natural and holistic form of healing.

Reiki was discovered by Mikao Usui in Japan at the turn of the twentieth century. He was a devout Christian who discovered the healing formula in a Buddhist text. This does not mean that Reiki practitioners have to be Christian or Buddhist: Reiki is non-denominational and distinct from other forms of spiritual healing. Dr Usui believed everyone has the potential to use healing energy, activated through an 'attunement' process, after which the person is able to give Reiki treatments to themselves and to others, subject to level and certification. There are now over 144 different types of Reiki being practised.

As you lie on the couch, fully clothed but comfortably dressed (no overly tight waistbands to distract your attention), the Reiki healer will commence channelling energy to dissolve blocks and encourage the free flow of energy and the state of balance in which the body's own healing processes are thought to work best. Sometimes you can feel a warmth or heat being generated through the healer's hands.

I always feel deeply relaxed and the sensation of not being alone, by which I mean a sense of oneness with others, a sense of connection between the visible and the invisible, and a deep sense of inner peace. In this state of deep relaxation, I normally fall asleep. I always feel great after a session, very happy, relaxed and full of energy.

On one occasion, I had come out of hospital after surgery and a Reiki master came to my home to treat me. This helped enormously with the side effects of the anaesthetic, and my road to recovery and healing was definitely speeded up. Reiki practitioners maintain that the body takes what it needs from the healing energies that are channelled for it. This healing energy does not treat only the physical condition. If you start thinking about painful memories, it may be that the body has decided it is time to address these, deal with them and move on in a happier state.

Further information

UK

Fidelma Spilsbury, reflexologist, Reiki and British Wheel of Yoga teacher, 254a Bath Road, Atworth, Melksham, Wiltshire, SN12 8JR. Email: fidelma. spilsbury@virgin.net

The lead body for Reiki practitioners in the UK is **The Reiki Council**, PO Box 1877, Andover SP11 9WT. Email: info@reikicouncil.org.uk. Website: www.reikicouncil.org.uk

Penny Brohn Cancer Care evidence-based information leaflet on healing: www.pennybrohncancercare.org/upload/docs/932/healing.pdf

Cancer Research UK: www.cancerhelp.org.uk/about-cancer/treatment/ complementary-alternative/therapies/reiki

US

Information on Reiki from the **National Center for Complementary and Alternative Medicine**: http://nccam.nih.gov/health/reiki

Reference

Living The Reiki Way: Traditional Principles For Living The Reiki Way by Penelope Quest. Piatkus (2010).

S is for Scans
X-rays and CT scans

Old-fashioned 'plain' X-rays have been around for over a century. They are good for identifying some body structures, most clearly bone. But many tissues absorb radiation to much the same extent. If a colon cancer produces secondary tumours in the liver, for example, an ordinary X-ray will generally not pick up the difference between healthy tissue and the cancer. Neither is it very good at pinpointing cancers in the brain. Sometimes it is possible to reveal more by injecting a radiation-opaque substance that becomes concentrated in the tumour. But a huge advance came with the development of 'computerized tomography' (CT) scanning which linked X-ray machines to sophisticated computers.

Instead of having one source of X-rays, a whole battery of X-ray sources and detectors is moved around the patient. An image is built up by pooling the information obtained from looking at the body from every angle, and very small and subtle differences can be detected. Another feature of this technique is that it provides cross-sectional views of the body – top to toe, and side to side – as if obtained by an optical bacon slicer. This allows the volume of a tumour to be calculated and greatly helps the assessment of response to treatment.

The CT procedure takes between 10 and 40 minutes, depending on the complexity of the scan. You should not eat or drink for a period – typically two hours – before the scan.

I had an 8.00 a.m. appointment and found that being deprived of my morning cup of coffee was torture. But a CT scan is not an experience to be anxious about – it is completely painless. I was given 900 ml of a mixture of lemon barley water and iodine, which wasn't too disgusting. This is to be drunk over a period of an hour so that it has time to travel through the body. I was also given an injection of 'contrast', a substance which makes the images clearer, though this is not always needed. There can be a slight tingling and metallic taste in the mouth (but this lasts

A
B
C
D
E
F
G
H
I
J
K
L
M
N
O
P
Q
R
S
T
U
V
W
X
Y
Z

only a few seconds) and a feeling of 'must have a pee' or 'going to pee involuntarily'. Thankfully this does not happen. And when I did later pass urine, I was surprised to see a fluorescent green, which is the body eliminating the iodine.

The scanner is best described as a large Polo mint. The patient lies flat on the scanning table which moves sedately through the 'mint' and out of the other side. I was given instructions to breathe in, out, and hold. Although the scanning table looks uncomfortable, I have managed to fall asleep.

MRI (Magnetic Resonance Imaging)

MRI does not use X-rays. Instead, the body is placed in an enormously strong magnetic field. Nuclei within the atoms that are the building blocks of our cells and tissues align themselves in a particular direction, like tiny bar magnets. There is then a brief pulse from a radiofrequency beam. This throws the nuclei out of alignment and, as they spin back, they emit signals at different frequencies, like small radio transmitters. Nuclei of different chemical elements emit different signals. Since different tissues are made up of different elements, plotting the source of the various kinds of radio signal builds up a picture of the inside of the body. MRI not only shows where different tissues are located but also provides information about the biochemical processes going on in those tissues, and these often reflect health or disease. MRI can also show the amount of blood flow to a particular area, which can be a useful indication of whether treatment is killing a tumour.

There is no radiation involved, so MRI is a safe scanning technique. However, because of the strong magnetic field, there is a pretty comprehensive form to complete prior to the scan – and it cannot be done when there are metal implants or a pacemaker. The downside of this scanner is that the whole body is enveloped by it. Instead of moving through a small tunnel, you have to lie in it. And this could feel claustrophobic. I had several of these scans and wondered why I always felt so sleepy for hours afterwards – until I was told that a Valium tablet was given as a matter of course. No wonder I was out like a light! I then declined the Valium. I can snooze wherever, even in the MRI scanner. But this may be rare because it is a noisy process. Some hospitals offer earplugs or headphones so that you can listen to music. The scan can last up to an hour so this is a good option.

Unlike a CT scan, no particular preparation is needed. You do not have to fast – unless otherwise instructed, as might be the case for an abdominal or pelvic scan. (For such scans, the patient is asked to drink large amounts of liquid – normally water. This helps in identification of the stomach and bowel.) An injection of contrast medium is usually given into a vein, to enhance the image. This can feel a touch cold going into the arm, but the sensation lasts only seconds. Otherwise it is all very straightforward.

PET (Positron Emission Tomography)

This is the newest form of scanning. It is special because it provides information not so much about structure as about function. More specifically, it shows the amount of metabolic activity at various points in the body. Just as with areas that are inflamed, there tends to be a lot of metabolic activity where there is a cancer, and these show up as hot-spots on a PET scan.

Cells that are very active use a lot of fuel, which, in the case of the body, is glucose. So a patient is injected with a form of glucose that has been labelled with a small dose of radioactivity. Cancer cells take up more radioactive glucose than normal tissue. And these areas of relatively high radioactivity are imaged by the scanner. The radioactivity then decays over a few hours.

PET scanning can be valuable in establishing how far certain tumours have spread. This is the case, for example, with some lung cancers, lymphomas and tumours of the oesophagus. It can also reveal how well a drug is working, and whether areas that appear abnormal on other scans are sites of active cancer or ones that have been killed by treatment. But in many patients there is no need for PET scanning. When a PET scan could prove useful, it may be necessary to travel to another hospital since not all centres have the facilities.

Ultrasound

Ultrasound is a way of looking at the soft organs in the body using high-frequency sound waves similar to those used in underwater sonar. Gel, usually fairly cold, is spread over the part of the body to be investigated and then a soft rounded probe is run over the gelled area, whether it be breast or abdomen. The sound waves emitted by the probe bounce back from surfaces within the body, creating an image on a monitor. Echoes are particularly strong where there is a change in the density of tissue, but images may be difficult to interpret without the benefit of other information. So ultrasound is often used to have a first look, prior to making further investigations with more sophisticated scanning techniques such as MRI or CT.

Bone scans

An X-ray gives a general picture of the condition of the bones but does not necessarily show up small areas where secondary tumours may have become established. So a bone scan might be suggested. This is a much more sensitive test. The patient is given a radioactive substance which is selectively taken up by areas of bone in which the metabolism is abnormal. But abnormal is not always cancerous – it could reflect arthritis or a sports injury, for example.

A small amount of blue-green dye which is mildly radioactive is injected into a vein, usually in the arm. You are asked to drink lots of water – in my case, seven cups – to encourage circulation. About three hours after the injection, you lie on a narrow trolley, strapped in place – nowhere to hide, nowhere to run! But no instruments of torture are immediately visible. In fact, this is a very easy experience, though you must keep still for a few minutes so that a clear picture is taken. It is very like a sophisticated X-ray. In my case, the X-ray 'plate' was lowered into place over me, but you often sit or stand in front of the scanner.

There is a bit of hanging around with a bone scan – the wait is three hours – so take a good book or your iPod, or something to do while you are there. I find concentrating on a book is hard under waiting-room conditions, so a friend gave me a small piece of tapestry to work on. I can't decide whether it should be a kneeler at my church or a footstool for my husband.

TOP TIPS

Radiation and chemical dyes are toxins that should be removed from the body forthwith after serving their purpose.

With X-rays and CT, the radiation dose is small but radiographers work with these machines all day and so operate them from a separate room. I found it quite amusing to communicate through a tannoy system, but you have to keep still – so laughing is to be avoided. Otherwise the radiographer will ask to do the whole process again.

As with most scans, patients having an MRI are given a hospital gown to change into. Clothes and other personal belongings are safely stored in an individual locker. The key of the cupboard is then put in the pocket of the gown. But because the MRI scan uses a strong magnetic field it's as well *to remember the key*!

Further information

UK

Cancer Research UK on different types of scans: www.cancerhelp.org.uk/about-cancer/tests/index.htm

US

American Cancer Society on different types of scans: www.cancer.org/Treatment/UnderstandingYourDiagnosis/ExamsandTestDescriptions/ImagingRadiologyTests/index

National Cancer Institute on imaging tests: http://imaging.cancer.gov/imaginginformation/cancerimaging

CancerGuide, 'Scan and Test Anxiety: A Guide for the Newcomer': http://cancerguide.org/scan_anxiety.html

S is for Screening

If cancer can be caught early, there is a much better chance of cure. Probably the best validated screening is that for cancer of the cervix (the neck of the womb). Strictly speaking, this programme is designed as prevention rather than early cure, since the aim is to detect abnormal cells that – if left untreated – are likely to develop into cancer. (It is thought that screening prevents 75% of cervix cancers in the UK.) But the principle is the same. Women aged 25–64 years are invited every 3–5 years to have the 'smear' test. Cells brushed from the cervix are examined in the lab to see if they show precancerous features. If they do, treatment is straightforward and can be done in an outpatient clinic.

Screening for breast cancer detects tumours when they are small and is described under 'M is for Mammogram'. Mammography is credited with saving many thousands of women's lives.

There is still debate about whether screening for prostate cancer would achieve the same result for men (see 'P is for Prostate Cancer'). Here, the standard test is not an X-ray but measurement in blood of a protein called prostate-specific antigen (PSA) which is usually abnormally high in men with prostate tumours. The problem is that levels are also high in some men who do not have prostate cancer; and in some men who do have the cancer, PSA levels are low. So PSA screening would unnecessarily worry some healthy men, and, in others, it would fail to detect the tumour. The first kind of mistaken result is called a false positive, and the second a false negative. The proportion of results which are false positives and false negatives are crucial when those with the job of looking after our health are deciding whether to introduce national screening programmes. And these are large projects: the cervix cancer programme screens four million women each year.

One such decision that has just been made in the UK is to introduce a screening programme designed to detect early bowel (or colorectal) cancer. This comes after research suggesting screening could reduce deaths from the disease by around 16%.

Bowel cancer is the third most common cancer in the UK, so that percentage reduction would amount to many lives saved. Region by region, people aged 60–69 years old are being asked to conduct a test at home that identifies small amounts of blood in faeces. Traces of blood do not necessarily mean that someone has bowel cancer, but they do show the need for further tests (see 'B is for Bowel (Colorectal) Cancer').

Further information
UK

NHS Cancer Screening Programmes: www.cancerscreening.nhs.uk

Cancer Research UK: www.cancerhelp.org.uk/about-cancer/causes-symptoms/screening-for-cancer

US

American Cancer Society screening guidelines: www.cancer.org/Healthy/FindCancerEarly/CancerScreeningGuidelines/american-cancer-society-guidelines-for-the-early-detection-of-cancer

S is for Shark Cartilage

The skeleton of a shark is made up almost entirely of cartilage, a sort of flexible connective and supporting tissue. Two features suggest that cartilage cells may produce substances that could be helpful in treating tumours. First, cartilage seems resistant to invasion by cancer cells. Second, cartilage does not have blood vessels. If this is because it secretes something that blocks blood vessel formation, that substance might also prevent a tumour from forming the blood vessels that it needs to grow.

Extracts of shark cartilage can be given as an injection under the skin, as an enema (fluid into the back passage) or taken orally in capsule form. There are anecdotal reports from cancer patients that suggest benefit. But shark (and cow) cartilage has been studied systematically in cancer patients and the results show no evidence that it is helpful. This is true both of the powdered shark cartilage sold as a food supplement and of a highly purified extract developed by a pharmaceutical company (and called Neovastat).

In an initial small study in patients with kidney cancer, Neovastat seemed to prolong survival. But this finding was not confirmed by a large randomized trial. And that was particularly disappointing since kidney cancer was a good choice of tumour in which to try the drug: kidney tumours have a lot of blood vessels, and any treatment that stops them developing should be helpful.

Neovastat was also used in a carefully controlled trial in 379 patients with advanced lung cancer. Those who had the shark cartilage added to their standard therapy did not survive longer than those who had standard therapy alone, and shark cartilage did not slow progression of the disease.

The first time I came across shark cartilage was when I had a distinctly dodgy cervical smear reading – this was the first time I had a house full of clean cupboards and told my husband where to find absolutely everything! Laser treatment was discussed and unfortunately – or fortunately – I had an awful cold, followed by the usual chest infection and so could not have the anaesthetic. In the meantime, Linda Crawford came to the rescue again. I took her homeopathic anti-cancer regime and went back to see my private gynaecologist (having sneakily had an NHS smear test which was clear) and asked to have the test privately again. This time it too was clear. My gynaecologist was suspicious and contacted the lab to ask whether there could have been a mistake in the initial test. He was told very definitely not: there was the full thickness of abnormal cells. So he then cross-questioned me, and I admitted to taking shark cartilage along with a host of other anti-cancer homeopathic remedies. He was surprised but, being highly experienced, not utterly in awe. Years later, when I was diagnosed with breast cancer of an aggressive kind that had already spread into the lymph nodes, I chose the orthodox path as my initial approach to treatment – there was no time to do otherwise.

Further information
UK

Cancer Research UK's information on shark cartilage: www.cancerhelp. org.uk/about-cancer/treatment/complementary-alternative/therapies/ shark-cartilage

Shark cartilage in capsule or powdered form is available from **The Nutri Centre** Tel: 0845 602 6744. Email admin@nutricentre.com. Website: www.nutricentre.com

US

Memorial Sloan-Kettering Cancer Center information on shark cartilage: www.mskcc.org/mskcc/html/69374.cfm

For **Lewis Gale Hospital's** information on shark cartilage, scroll down to 'Natural and Alternative Treatments' on the main menu of the website and click on 'Herbs and Supplements'. Then find 'Shark cartilage' in the A–Z list: www.alleghanyregional.com/healthcontent.asp?page=contentselection/condensedmainindex

References

Sharks Still Don't Get Cancer: The Continuing Story of Shark Cartilage Therapy by I. William Lane and Linda Comac. Avery (1996).

'Chemoradiotherapy with or without AE-941 [Neovastat] in stage III non-small cell lung cancer: A randomized phase III trial' by C. Lu and colleagues. *Journal of the National Cancer Institute* 2010, volume 102, pages 859–865.

S is for Spiritual (Incorporating Soul Work)

See also 'M is for Mind, Body, Spirit and Healing'

I cannot exactly say when I became aware that I had a spiritual side. I had an ectopic pregnancy when I was 30 and nearly died on the operating table according to the doctor. I think I knew that because I had been outside my body watching the panic going on around my physical body below. Then came the light which was so attractive and I felt as if I was at a party – not of strangers, but of really good friends who I hadn't seen for a while; but we were all delighted to see each other again. There was a feeling of deep comradeship, of something more glorious than being human, because there was none of the nonsense of humanity, the petty jealousies, the one-upmanship. This was pure 'love thy friend and neighbour', unadulterated. Then came the question, would I like to go towards the light? And I said, 'No, I must get back to earth. I have got things to do.' The next day I came round in the ward and to this day I have not known what on earth was so important that I had to do. For the next 18 years I completely ignored this experience and lived my life as a director of a property investment and development company in the City. The last thing I thought of was anything at all spiritual. The diagnosis of cancer and the spiritual turning point collided, or coincided.

Probably the most positive aspect of a diagnosis of cancer is that you have absolute permission to look at, delve into and investigate your own life's purpose – your soul's contract. It was sad that it took a diagnosis of cancer, hanging over my head like Damocles' sword, to make me want to address this. Many people progressing through their physical life think automatically of the wider context, the universe and God. They do not need cancer to concentrate their minds on the greater scheme of things. But for this little party person – tripping through life, working inordinately hard and playing even harder – there was no time to stand and stare, no time even to smell the roses and no time to acknowledge there is an inner voice, let alone listen to it. I had 48 years of catapulting through life. How do you bring all this to a halt? A diagnosis of cancer – perfect.

On Thursday I was diagnosed with cancer; on Sunday I was in church. It was All Saints' Day – not that I would have known – and Father Andrew was explaining to the children about Gabriel the messenger, St Raphael the healer and St Michael the fighter. I thought vaguely that I could do with the help of Raphael and Michael. The sermon continued with 'If thine eye offends thee, cut it out' – at which point I was completely convinced I should have the surgery. You have to remember here the shocked and vulnerable state of someone just diagnosed with cancer.

That Sunday afternoon, my wonderful friend Linda Crawford came to see me armed with her biofeedback and alpha machines. She was one of the four people who knew of my diagnosis. But she did not know I had run off to church. As a healer, she is not tied to one religion like me. Having spent a good hour treating me, she was standing on the doorstep to leave when she said, 'I nearly forgot, I was thinking about you earlier and I bought you these.' I took from her three votives. They were Gabriel the messenger of hope, St Raphael the healer and St Michael the warrior. 'If you wake in the night and can't sleep,' she said, 'put these under your pillow.' They remain with me four years later and remind me that this was a simply HUGE message. I was absolutely not alone, and I have never felt alone, and – sometimes when I least expect it – I am reminded: I literally bump into Michael, Raphael and Gabriel.

It was while undergoing chemotherapy that something extraordinary happened. I changed, and as I changed so did the people around me. I went to Penny Brohn Cancer Care in Bristol (formerly Bristol Cancer Help Centre; see 'P is for Penny Brohn Cancer Care') and had a transformational experience which set me on the path to spiritual growth. The secret to slowing me down so that my soul could get back on track and fulfil my life's purpose was – yes – more cancer.

Bristol unlocked my spirit and let it fly. Nothing was impossible, and everything was possible. I knew (and this in retrospect has been confirmed) that my life would be about representing others less able to represent themselves, people less articulate, less punchy, or just with more commitments. Amongst this group there were the connoisseurs of cancer, the sacrificial lambs, and me, the fighter, in need of constant healing, but with something to say – a message – on behalf of others.

It became known that I welcomed fielding phone calls from people just diagnosed, or those who felt there was no hope left, and I knew the book I could write was much needed. I telephoned a friend, Delissa Needham, whom I had met in Antigua quite by chance, and over lunch she formatted the shape of the book, the title, the strategy – all I had to do was to start writing.

On another occasion I vividly recollect Father Andrew talking to the children in the church about St Patrick and his life, and how, because of the death of Jesus, we all have the Holy Spirit within us. THIS WAS THE MESSAGE – if we can put ourselves in the position of complete peace and empty our minds of all the chitter-chatter, we can hear the still, small voice of calm, have tangible communication and obtain guidance within our lives.

TOP TIP

The inner voice is the voice of the spirit.

Further information

UK

Hospitals Chaplaincy Council, Church House, Great Smith Street, London SW1P 3AZ. Tel: 020 7898 1892. Website: www.nhs-chaplaincy-spiritualcare.org.uk/theroleofthechaplain.htm

National Federation of Spiritual Healers Tel: 01604 603247. Website: www.nfsh.org.uk

The College of Psychic Studies, 16 Queensberry Place, London SW7 2EB. Tel: 020 7589 3292. Website: www.collegeofpsychicstudies.co.uk

Penny Brohn Cancer Care evidence-based information sheet on healing: www.pennybrohncancercare.org/upload/docs/932/healing.pdf

US

American Cancer Society on spirituality and prayer: www.cancer.org/ Treatment/TreatmentsandSideEffects/ComplementaryandAlternative Medicine/MindBodyandSpirit/spirituality-and-prayer

National Cancer Institute on spirituality in cancer care: www.cancer.gov/ cancertopics/pdq/supportivecare/spirituality/Patient

Episode 7 in *The Seven Levels of Healing* by Dr Jeremy Geffen is connecting with spirit, the profound sense of oneness or belonging, the spiritual dimension of life we all share, the source of healing. See **Caring4Cancer**: www.caring4cancer.com/go/cancer/videos/seven-level-of-healing-web-vidoes.htm?moviename=/Caring4HealthAssets/videos/SLH/Level7/ Level7.flv&title=Level+7:+Nature+of+Spirit

References

Defy Gravity: How to Heal Beyond the Boundaries of Ordinary Reason by Caroline M. Myss. Hay House (2009).

Wherever You Go, There You Are: Mindfulness Meditation for Everyday Life by Jon Kabat-Zin. Piatkus (2004).

Anti-cancer: A New Way of Life by David Servan-Schreiber. Michael Joseph (2008).

Sacred Contracts: Awakening Your Divine Potential by Caroline M. Myss. Bantam Books (2002).

S is for Statistics

For me, too much of the cancer journey is expressed in those dreadful, impersonal statistics – the percentage chances of surviving after the operation, with or without chemotherapy/ radiotherapy/drugs, etc. for one year, two years, five years and so on.

I am not a statistic and neither are you. We are both individuals. Statistics are just mathematical averages. They cannot take into account the myriad of personal circumstances that make me/you different from everybody else. Maybe it is worth trying to find out what our chances are, particularly as a means of choosing between different kinds of treatment available. But statistics are historical – they are backward – not forward-looking. If they do indicate the odds, then it is up to you to beat them.

TOP TIP

You're a person, not a bloody statistic!

Further information

Stephen Jay Gould wrote an excellent essay on cancer statistics entitled 'The Median Isn't the Message'. Many cancer patients have found his thoughts useful. Link to an online copy of the essay: http://fog.ccsf.edu/~abair/median.pdf

If you are interested in understanding more about statistics, a patient advocacy group **Patients Against Lymphoma** has put together a primer on statistics for cancer patients: www.lymphomation.org/CAM-evaluating.htm#terms

S is for Supplements

It is said that a balanced diet provides all the nutrients, minerals and vitamins the body requires without need for supplements. Do we believe this?

Various assumptions have been made, which do not include the fast-food breakfast consisting of a coffee on the hoof and the fast-food lunch – if there is lunch at all – of sandwich, packet of crisps and a Kit Kat. How much education do we need to replace the sandwich with a rice cake and oily fish; the crisps with a packet of nuts, seeds and dried fruit; the Kit Kat with an apple? (The apple, in the hope it has not been sprayed with – and absorbed – all sorts of carcinogens.)

Another assumption is that you have had time to study what supplements you *might* need. And I suggest you probably have not – until, that is, you have a diagnosis of cancer, when you,

A
B
C
D
E
F
G
H
I
J
K
L
M
N
O
P
Q
R
S
T
U
V
W
X
Y
Z

like me, think maybe now is the time. Better late than never, but how much better it would have been if you or I had thought of this before.

In my case, I would enjoy and think about food if I was having a social dinner, but otherwise it would be convenient and quick refuelling with no concern about what my mother called 'goodness'. Realizing that I was in for the long haul in terms of cancer treatments, my views on food, nutrition and the role of supplements completely changed. I realized I needed to be 'match fit' and as strong as I could to withstand both the disease and its treatment.

There are, of course, supplements and supplements. The cheaper supplements might not have the same natural product, and have more preservatives, colourings and perhaps even artificial sweeteners. If you shop at a specialist centre (such as the Nutricentre at the Hale Clinic in London, or Penny Brohn Cancer Care – formerly Bristol Cancer Help Centre – in Bristol), there are pharmacists with expert information to help you make an informed decision. Most centres have mail-order facilities.

(See also 'A is for Antioxidant Vitamins and Minerals'; 'F is for Folic Acid'; 'V is for Vitamins'.)

Further information
UK

The Nutri Centre, Unit 3, Kendal Court, Kendal Avenue, London W3 0RU. Tel: 0845 602 6744. Email: admin@nutricentre.com. Website: www.nutricentre.com For your nearest store: www.nutricentre.com/t-ourstores.aspx. For any nutritional queries contact the Nutri Centre's nutritionists on 020 7436 5122 (or +44 20 8752 8450 if outside the UK).

Penny Brohn Cancer Care, Chapel Pill Lane, Bristol BS20 0HH. Tel: 01275 370 112. *The Bristol Approach to Supplements: A Guide to How to Maintain Optimal Nutrient Levels whilst Living with Cancer* (2010) downloadable from www.pennybrohncancercare.org/upload/docs/932/pbcc_supplement_guidelines_2010.pdf. Also visit: www.shopatpennybrohn.com

US

Three resources with excellent information on herbs and supplements:

Medline Plus, a service of the National Institute of Health: www.nlm.nih.gov/medlineplus/druginfo/herb_All.html

Lewis Gale Hospital website. Scroll down to 'Natural and Alternative Treatments' on the main menu, click on 'NAT index', then browse through the 'Herbs and Supplements' section: www.alleghanyregional.com/health content.asp?page=contentselection/condensedmainindex

Memorial Sloan-Kettering Cancer Center, 'About Herbs, botanicals and other products': www.mskcc.org/mskcc/html/11570.cfm

In the United States, supplements are not regulated. Several reputable independent groups have begun testing products to ensure that they contain what they claim and are not contaminated. **Consumer Reports Health** is one of these groups: www.consumerreports.org/health/natural-health.htm; **ConsumerLab** is another: www.consumerlab.com. Both are subscription services but worth the money if you are interested in purchasing quality supplements.

S is for Surgery

When a cancer is detected before it has time to spread to other parts of the body, an operation can cure the disease. Once and for all. Surgery cures more cancers than any other therapy. Yet it sometimes does not receive the credit it deserves.

Cutting out the cancer is the traditional method of treatment when the tumour is all in one place, not too large, and easy to get to. The tumour is taken where possible with 'wide margins', which is to say areas around the tumour which look to have no cancer but might contain the odd escaped cancerous cell. This 'margin' goes to the pathology lab where it is examined (see 'H is for Histology') and either judged to be cancer-free, or not. If the margin is found to contain more cancer cells, the recommendation may be more surgery or other treatment such as chemotherapy or radiotherapy. Sometimes the tumour is removed along with the surrounding lymph nodes, often in one piece.

Advances in anaesthetics, blood transfusion and the use of blood products, surgical techniques and antibiotics have all made it possible to do more complicated surgery where necessary while maintaining the safety of operations.

A
B
C
D
E
F
G
H
I
J
K
L
M
N
O
P
Q
R
S
T
U
V
W
X
Y
Z

As well as removing all of the cancer, or as much as can safely be achieved, surgery has a role in the relief of symptoms. A notable example is the insertion of tubes or expanding coils (stents) to relieve blockages. This can be done in many areas of the body such as the throat, the bronchi leading to the lungs or the bile duct leading to the bowel. Surgery can also help in pain relief.

S is for Symptoms

Symptoms are as individually felt as the cancer. Some people suffer pain and that must be professionally handled to ensure the best possible quality of life. Some people suffer extreme tiredness which is further fuelled by anxiety and depression. This is a difficult cycle to break, again requiring professional help. And there are many symptoms such as mouth sores and lack of appetite caused by chemotherapy or radiotherapy.

For four years, apart from surgery, I had only odd twinges of pain, lasting seconds, which I have breathed my way out of. Only once did pain stop me from doing what I wanted to do. I was changing to go out and the 'twinge' was so dramatic that I vomited, and I rang to cancel my appointment. I was then fine, and to this day I do not know if the pain was associated with cancer or some sort of violent food poisoning. And that is the point: if you have cancer, you associate all and everything that happens with either the cancer or the drugs.

I have tended to steer away from any literature about symptoms, because it is in itself depressing. All possible symptoms are listed. The likelihood is you will not get them all. Some of them you will have only slightly, and you may experience none. I really do not want to dwell on all the symptoms I MIGHT have. I would rather plan all the fun I CAN have. But 'symptoms' of tiredness, whether suffered or not, are a great excuse to watch the afternoon movie on TV, have a snooze after lunch and chomp through the odd box of chocs. If you come out in spots, you can blame the drugs!

TOP TIP

Don't let your symptoms get on top of you – if you feel they are, get professional help quickly so you can enjoy life.

Further information

UK

Cancer Research UK: www.cancerhelp.org.uk/coping-with-cancer/coping-physically/pain/index.htm, and www.cancerhelp.org.uk/coping-with-cancer/coping-emotionally/talking-about-cancer/what-you-can-do

Macmillan Cancer Support for information on treatment types and possible side effects: www.macmillan.org.uk/Cancerinformation/Cancertreatment/Treatmenttypes

References

Coping Successfully with Pain (Overcoming Common Problems) by Neville Shone. Sheldon Press (2002).

Beating Stress, Anxiety and Depression: Groundbreaking Ways to Help You Feel Better by Jane Plant and Janet Stephenson. Piatkus Books (2008).

A
B
C
D
E
F
G
H
I
J
K
L
M
N
O
P
Q
R
S
T
U
V
W
X
Y
Z

T is for Tai Chi

Tai Chi is often described as 'meditation in motion', or, it has been said, 'medication in motion'. There is growing evidence that this mind–body practice, which originated in China as a martial art, has value in treating or preventing many health problems. Qigong practice (see 'Q is for Qigong'), principally sitting and standing meditation, provides the energetic foundation of Tai Chi as both work with the breath (*qi* or *chi*), intention and focus. However, in addition to the energy balancing and strengthening practices that Tai Chi has in common with Qigong, Tai Chi movements involve either expressing force (internal power/energy) or directing force. As a martial art, students training with partners learn how to sense the direction of an attack and, to quote the classic teaching of the art, how 'to use one ounce to deflect a thousand pounds'. This training is referred to as 'pushing hands'.

According to legend, Zhang San Feng, a Taoist monk who had already mastered Shaolin Boxing, caught sight of a crane fighting a snake. Intrigued by the yielding, smooth evasion and darting counter-attacks of both creatures, he was inspired to develop a new form of boxing which would also embody the natural philosophy of the Tao – in essence the 'way' of nature and the universe.

Legend aside, in the middle of the eighteenth century, Yang Luchan – who had popularized the Chen family 'soft boxing' style in Henan Province – went to Beijing. There he taught the art, in a modified form, to the Manchu court, the last ruling dynasty of China. This Yang school of boxing was destined to become the most popular form of Tai Chi. It is characterized by large, smooth and flowing movements and, uncharacteristically for martial arts as understood today, avoids strenuous over-exertion. Walk in any park in China, just as day is dawning, and there will be hundreds of people performing graceful, almost balletic, movements such as 'white crane spreads its wings', while breathing deeply and slowly.

In Chinese medicine, doctors teach their patients to master the flow of energy in their own bodies. Through combined mental and physical practice involving relaxation, focusing on the breath and releasing all thoughts, they teach patients to find the spot in their body or 'dantian' point, just below the navel, where their *chi* begins. By concentrating on the ball of energy, it is possible to learn to move it and clear energy blocks in the body.

Tai Chi promotes natural and correct posture; the cardiovascular system is gently exercised as the positions the student adopts strengthen the body in general and the legs in particular. A series of slow focused and deliberate movements, practised as 'forms', improves balance and promotes confidence, but also greatly reduces the risk of injury from other activities. Studies illustrate the many physical and mental benefits of Tai Chi in the recovery from and management of cancer and recommend more extensive research. Benefits include an enhanced immune response, improved digestion, sleep and respiration, and relief from pain, depression, stress and anxiety. When the student holds the spine in correct alignment, turning and moving the waist, the parasympathetic nervous system – the body's restraint on the flight or fight syndrome – is stimulated. This decreases heart rate and dilates the blood vessels, improving circulation. The mind remains calm as the person becomes so absorbed by the practice that all worries are forced aside, being replaced by a state of alert relaxation.

In the West, Tai Chi is becoming increasingly popular as its extensive health benefits are recognized. World Tai Chi and Qigong Day was started in the late 1990s by author Bill Douglas as a way to introduce people to the profound healing and health maintenance benefits of Tai Chi and Qigong. The event has grown into a worldwide phenomenon, taking place in over 60 countries. It starts at 10 a.m. in the earliest time zone on the last Saturday every April, and is said to flow as a gentle wave across the entire planet.

A B C D E F G H I J K L M N O P Q R S T U V W X Y Z

A gentle practice for those dealing with illness, Tai Chi is accessible to all, including those who have given their best years to other sports and are now looking for a less physically demanding challenge and strengthening exercise. When asked by a student, 'What is the most important reason to study Tai Chi Chuan?', Master Cheng Man Ching is said to have replied, 'The most important reason is that when you finally reach the place where you understand what life is about, you'll have the health to enjoy it.'

TOP TIP

There are many instructional DVDs available and videos on the internet, but nothing compares with finding a teacher and learning from a master. Take the time to go and simply watch some classes in your area. They will probably all have a different feel, so study the pupils, the way they move and learn about their experiences. To begin with at least, it is important to feel comfortable in your surroundings so that you can really let go of your preconceptions and inhibitions and try something new. The Chinese say, 'When the time is right the teacher will appear.'

Further information
UK

Tai Chi Finder Ltd, 21 The Avenue, London E11 2EE. Tel: 020 8819 2767. Website: www.taichifinder.co.uk

Taiji Qigong Foundation: www.uktqf.co.uk

US

The online journal of the **American Tai Chi and Qigong Association** includes a searchable database of providers by state: www.americantaichi.net

Some major cancer centres offer Tai Chi classes as part of their integrative medicine programmes. Tai Chi classes that are free for cancer survivors are often offered at support centres such as **Gilda's Club**: www.gildasclub.org, and **The Wellness Community**: www.thewellnesscommunity.org

References
'A randomized trial of Tai Chi for Fibromyalgia' by Chenchen Wang and colleagues. *New England Journal of Medicine* August 2010.

Eternal Spring: Taijiquan, Qi Gong, and the Cultivation of Health, Happiness and Longevity by Michael W. Acton. Singing Dragon (2009).

Chen: Living Taijiquan in the Classical Style by Master Jan Silberstorff. Singing Dragon (2009).

Tai Chi For Health by Zhenglie Chen (author) and Liming Yue (translator). Chen Style Tai Chi Centre (2005).

T is for Tamoxifen

Tamoxifen was a breakthrough for women with breast tumours which grow in response to oestrogen. By blocking the growth-stimulating effect of this hormone, tamoxifen slows the progress of disease and gains time for women whose breast cancer has spread. In women whose cancer seems to be confined to the breast, taking tamoxifen after surgery (usually for five years) improves their chances of staying free of the disease. Used with this aim in mind (see 'A is for Adjuvant Therapy'), tamoxifen has saved tens of thousands of lives. In fact, the University of Oxford Clinical Trials Unit estimated ten years ago that the tamoxifen then being taken by around a million women worldwide was saving 20,000 lives a year.

Its use does increase the risk that a cancer will develop in the lining of the womb (though this is not a common cancer), and tamoxifen also increases the risk of deep vein thrombosis and of stroke. But this may be counterbalanced at least to some extent by a beneficial effect on the heart due to reduced levels of cholesterol in the blood. And the overall benefit of tamoxifen far outweighs its risks.

Aromatase inhibitors (see 'A is for Aromatase Inhibitors') are a newer class of drugs effective against oestrogen positive tumours, but tamoxifen continues to play a major role in treatment. The side effects of aromatase inhibitors and tamoxifen are different, and for many women tamoxifen may be preferable.

Further information
UK

Cancer Research UK: www.cancerhelp.org.uk/about-cancer/treatment/cancer-drugs/tamoxifen

US

National Cancer Institute: www.cancer.gov/cancertopics/factsheet/Therapy/tamoxifen

American Cancer Society: www.cancer.org/Treatment/TreatmentsandSideEffects/GuidetoCancerDrugs/tamoxifen

T is for Thermography

Thermography – or DIT (digital infrared thermal imaging) – is a technique that produces images based on the emission of non-visible, infrared radiation. Since the amount of this radiation produced by objects depends on their temperature, thermography – as its name implies – is essentially a means of mapping differences in heat.

Tumours tend to have a high rate of metabolism and co-opt the blood supply they need to keep growing. So they are often warmer than surrounding healthy tissue. The hope is that ultra-sensitive thermography cameras can be used to detect breast tumours at a stage even earlier than can be picked up by mammography. The procedure is non-invasive, safe, and does not use radiation or any sort of compression to obtain an image.

It is thought that breast cancers can be a decade or so in growing to a size that can be felt. And precancerous changes will have existed for even longer. If it were possible to detect abnormal growth in its very earliest stages, there might be a role for homeopathic or naturopathic support of the immune system to get the problem under control using the body's own resources, perhaps with the help of a vaccine (see 'V is for Vaccines').

Further information
UK

The Chiron Clinic, 104 Harley Street, London W1G 7JD. Tel: 020 72244 622. Website: www.chironclinic.com

Cancer Research UK: www.cancerhelp.org.uk/about-cancer/cancer-questions/thermography-or-heat-mapping

US

Breast Thermography.org constantly update their library of articles: www.breastthermography.org

American College of Thermology: www.thermologyonline.org/patients_overview.htm

T is for Traditional Chinese Medicine

The *Yellow Emperor's Classic of Internal Medicine* is the first record of the teachings which form the foundation of Traditional Chinese Medicine (TCM). Written between 200 BC and AD 100 in the form of a discussion between the author and his doctor about medicine, health, lifestyle and nutrition, the Yellow Emperor emphasized three of the ideals of Taoist philosophy: balance, harmony and moderation in all things.

Traditional Chinese Medicine is holistic in its approach and includes acupuncture, diet, herbal therapy, meditation, massage and Qigong and Tai Chi exercises (see related sections). For thousands of years it has been used to prevent, diagnose and treat disease. According to the principles of all Chinese medicine, health exists when the body is in balance and vital energy is freely flowing along its 20 meridians (channels). The term 'vital energy' refers to *qi* (see 'Q is for Qigong'), which is inherited, sourced from the digestion of food and absorbed from the air we breathe. The term 'balance' refers to *yin* and *yang*, the opposite but complementary forces whose perfect balance within the body is essential for well-being. TCM aims to restore the body's balance and harmony between the forces of *yin* and *yang*, which can deplete or block *qi* and cause 'dis-ease'.

Representing one of the most profound theories of Taoist philosophy, the *yin yang* symbol is one of the best-known life symbols. The white *yang* blends into the black *yin* symbolizing dependent opposing forces that flow in a natural cycle, always seeking balance. Each contains the seed of the other, hence the black spot of *yin* in the white *yang* and vice versa. The relationship between *yin* and *yang* is best described in terms of sunlight playing over a mountain and valley. *Yin* is the dark area in the shadow of the mountain, while *yang* is the brightly lit side. As the sun moves across the sky, *yin* and *yang* gradually trade places, revealing what was obscured, and obscuring what was revealed, darkness yielding to brightness and brightness to darkness. *Yin* and *yang* are two aspects of a single reality, mirrored in all matter.

Yin and *yang* are applied in TCM to explain all aspects of physiology, anatomy and pathology. In diagnosis, by characterizing symptoms of disease, it is possible to determine if a condition is mostly *yin* or *yang* and choose an appropriate balancing treatment. *Yang* conditions are exterior, excess and hot, and pertain to hyperactive and functional disease, whilst *yin* conditions are interior, deficient and cold, and relate to degeneration, hypo-activity and organic disease. This metaphorical view of the human body, based on observations of nature, is also expressed in the system of *Five Elements*: fire, earth, metal, water and wood. These categories represent the qualities of and interaction between everything in the universe. In TCM, the organs are seen as complex systems including not only their anatomical entity and role in the body, but also their corresponding emotional function. These relationships reflect the interaction of natural elements where one element supports or inhibits the function of another. For example, fire melts metal, water douses fire, wood promotes fire, fire promotes earth, and so on. In the body, the organs share the same relationships. For example, the heart controls the lungs and the kidneys control the heart.

These dynamic interactions enable all the organ systems to work as one harmonious greater system. If their relationships are good, a state of wellness prevails; if any of the relationships become unbalanced, health problems result. The TCM practitioner uses the qualities of the *Five Elements* to understand disharmony and restore balance. Having identified a pattern of disharmony in the body, the practitioner will recommend the appropriate herbal remedies, treatment and exercise, diet and/or lifestyle changes to correct the relationship between the elements and balance the body's *yin* and *yang*.

Diet is considered to be a major factor in cancer prevention and recurrence. Many foods have been found to contain anti-cancer agents. Research on soya beans and soya food products indicates that genistein, a type of phytoestrogen, can block the signal that triggers normal cells to become cancerous and scientists speculate that it may even be used as a cancer treatment. Recommended in TCM for their anti-cancer, immune-boosting or anti-inflammatory properties are green tea (see 'C is for Catechins'), shiitake mushrooms, garlic, kelp, ginger, carrots, cabbage and cauliflower.

Herbal medicine involves the ingestion of tinctures, powders and decoctions of plant materials. Chinese herbalists rarely prescribe a single herb to treat a condition. Instead, they create formulas containing various combinations of herbs to correct deficiencies or excesses of *qi* and balance the body. A symptom is not treated in isolation but as part of a syndrome. If a herb is considered toxic in its effect on the body, others are given to support the body and neutralize side effects. The herbs are classified under the *Five Elements* according to the remedial action of their taste – sour, bitter, sweet, pungent and salty – and their opposing *yin* and *yang* qualities of hot and cold. Cancer patients are prescribed sweet and warming astragalus during chemotherapy to support the immune system and decrease the toxic effect. Other immune system enhancing herbs are ginseng, cinnamon, Chinese foxglove root, turtle seed, *Cordyceps sinensis*, reishi, peony and licorice. To relieve toxicity, honeysuckle, forsythia, tangerine peel, lycii fruit and ligustrum seed are widely used.

Over 50% of prescription drugs are derived from chemicals first identified in plants. Examples include treatments for malaria using the leaves of *Artemisia annua* and medication to help fight cancer, dementia and heart disease from the magnolia plant, which has been used in TCM for over 5,000 years. The Western scientific community increasingly recognizes the potential of products from medicinal plants used for centuries in Traditional Chinese Medicine.

Taxanes, originally discovered in the 1960s in the leaves and bark of the Pacific yew tree native to North America, are a key constituent in chemotherapy regimes used with prostate, breast, ovarian and lung cancers. The Chinese yew tree, *Taxus chinensis*, now a protected species, is today a reliable source of high-quality natural paclitaxel. Other chemotherapy treatments are derived from the periwinkle plant, a source of vinca drugs, and the Chinese happy tree, containing camptothecin, and highly valued for its potential chemo-preventive role.

In China, the vast majority of cancer patients use Traditional Chinese Medicine along with conventional therapies. In the UK, more cancer patients are discovering the benefits of TCM in complementary care. Please refer to your doctor for advice.

Further information
UK

College of Integrated Chinese Medicine (information, clinic, training, register of practitioners), 19 Castle Street, Reading, Berkshire RG1 7SB. Tel: 0118 950 8880. Website: www.reading-berkshire.co.uk/college-of-integrated-chinese-medicine

Register of Chinese Herbal Medicine, Office 5, 1 Exeter Street, Norwich NR2 4QB. Tel: 01603 623994. Email: herbmed@rchm.co.uk. Website: www.rchm.co.uk

US

National Certification Commission for Acupuncture and Chinese Medicine (help in locating a certified provider): www.nccaom.org/find/index.html

American Chinese Medicine Association: www.americanchinesemedicineassociation.org

Traditional Chinese Medicine Association & Alumni, Inc. (TCMAA): www.tcmaa.org

Reference
Traditional Chinese Medicine Approaches To Cancer: Harmony in the Face of the Tiger by Henry McGrath. Singing Dragon (2009).

V is for Vaccines

We have all experienced vaccination against infections. The basic principle is that a small amount of the disease-causing agent (be it tuberculosis, measles or flu) is injected to stimulate the immune system to recognize the disease and fight it. The aim of a cancer vaccine is similar: it seeks to stimulate the immune system to recognize and destroy abnormal cells.

Over a hundred years ago it was noticed that patients who survived a severe infection sometimes had spontaneous resolution of their cancer. This led William Coley, a New York surgeon, to try to simulate the effects of infection (including development of a high fever) by giving patients a mixture of killed bacteria. This became known as 'Coley's toxins' and was arguably the first cancer vaccine. Although occasionally effective, there were patients who died from treatment, and Coley's toxins fell into disuse.

Since then, a wide variety of cancer vaccines has been investigated, particularly for melanoma. Melanoma is one of the relatively few types of tumour (another being kidney cancer) which is reasonably immunogenic, which means you can detect that the immune system is trying to get to grips with it. Some good responses were reported anecdotally, but melanoma vaccines have not improved survival when tested rigorously in randomized trials. Over the last few years it has become clear that cancers in general can suppress the immune system by secreting a variety of substances and that boosting the immune response may be a helpful approach to treatment. So we have seen vaccines used against many types of tumour.

The first vaccines to show some clinical benefit in randomized trials were in colorectal and renal cancer. Both vaccines had to be prepared from tissue taken from the patients' cancers, a labour-intensive procedure that could not be widely applied. Recently, controlled trials of Provenge in advanced prostate cancer have provided the first confirmation that a vaccine can significantly prolong survival. On average, men given the active vaccine survived for 26 months – four months longer than men given a placebo vaccine. This is not a huge difference, but it proves the point that vaccines can alter the course of the disease; and Provenge is now approved for use in the United States. (See also 'P is for Prostate Cancer'.)

This vaccine has to be manufactured using cells taken from each patient's blood. But we are now also making vaccines using artificial antigens or immune-stimulatory components. So we should be able to develop widely applicable 'off the shelf' vaccines rather than having to tailor each one to the characteristics of a particular patient.

In the UK, the Cancer Vaccine Institute, headed by Professor Angus Dalgleish, has been conducting trials of a number of different vaccines, mainly in melanoma and prostate cancer. These trials show that a significant number of patients obtain clinical benefit from vaccination but, just as importantly, many do not. The focus now is on finding how to identify those who will benefit so they can be selected for early treatment. In parallel with this, efforts are being made to develop ways of reducing resistance to vaccination, perhaps by using drugs that take the brakes off the body's immune system or cytokines (see 'I is for Interleukin and Interferon') that can expand the number of T cells.

Doctors have noticed that patients who have had immunotherapy tend to respond better to other treatments (such as radiation) than those who have not had their immune systems stimulated. This suggests that vaccines will come to be used in combination with other anti-cancer therapies.

What has been said above relates to vaccines as a way of treating cancer. It should not be forgotten that there are already two vaccines very effective in *preventing* the disease. A vaccine against the hepatitis B virus, which is a major cause of liver cancer, has been saving many lives, especially in Asia, for many years. And vaccines that prevent infection with genital wart viruses that cause cancer of the cervix have just been introduced.

TOP TIP
From a patient's point of view, the great news about vaccines is that they have few or no side effects and therefore one can lead a 'normal life' while the body silently fights the cancer from within.

Further information
UK

Cancer Vaccine Institute, Haysmacintyre, Fairfax House, 15 Fulwood Place, London, WC1V 6AY. Principal: Professor Angus Dalgleish, Bsc (Hons) MD FRACPath FRACP FRCP FMedSci. Website:: www.cancervaccine.org.uk

Macmillan Cancer Support: www.macmillan.org.uk/Cancerinformation/Cancertreatment/Treatmenttypes/Biologicaltherapies/Vaccines.aspx

US

National Cancer Institute: www.cancer.gov/cancertopics/factsheet/Therapy/cancer-vaccines

American Cancer Society: www.cancer.org/Treatment/TreatmentsandSideEffects/TreatmentTypes/immunotherapy/immunotherapy-cancer-vaccines

EU

Dr Thomas Nesselhut, Institute of Tumour Therapy, Duderstadt, Germany. Tel: 0049 5527 99710

V is for Visualization

Some people find visualisation extremely useful, and I found it particularly helpful when I was faced with chemotherapy. I had a major battle convincing myself I should have chemo (see 'C is for Chemotherapy'). It was an intellectual problem: how can this be a therapy when it kills all fast-dividing cells – the good with the bad – and compromises the very immune system we rely on for our long-term survival?

I thought it was important to believe that chemotherapy would help my survival. Otherwise, it would be unlikely to do so. But I was also extremely anxious about having injected into my veins a pink substance I

had heard was not dissimilar to industrial bleach. The nurses wear gloves in case any of this particularly toxic substance splashes onto their hands.

I did make the right decision and had the chemotherapy, but I armed myself with some relaxation, meditation and visualization classes and a tape from Jan de Vries for breathing exercises.

Having done my preparation, I started practising visualization as soon as I had my first injection. I imagined the pink fluid as the colour of unconditional love. I visualized it entering my veins to seek out the naughty, child-like, out-of-control cancer cells zooming around my body trying to find a new home since their previous one, my right breast, was no longer available. And I visualized the cells being escorted to my liver and kidneys and off the premises.

Other people have more dramatic visualizations such as crocodiles appearing out of swamps, munching the cancer cells and exiting through the breath – crocodile breath. Every good visualization must have an exit route for the cancer cells. One visualization I heard of sounded more like a scene from a James Bond film. The white cells were dressed in arctic fighting gear and were marching up the body from the foot (presumably where the chemotherapy was being injected through a cannula). They were on the hunt for cancer cells, black spots in the snow. I'd like to know what happened next. Hope the good guys won.

As a child, when faced with something awful like sea sickness on car ferries, I used to imagine that I was actually doing my favourite thing, which was riding horses, and each lurch (or wave) was a jump. As a child I probably imagined; as an adult I visualize – but the technique is just as effective! I can become completely engrossed thinking about new garden designs while having an injection, or being scanned.

Visualization of a positive nature, such as being fit and well and doing the things that you most enjoy, reinforces the messages to the body on a cellular level. Although it might sound far-fetched, there is scientific evidence that patients can strengthen their immune system's response to cancer by using this methodology (see 'P is for Psychoneuroimmunology and the Power of Positive Thought').

TOP TIP

Let your imagination run wild! Visualize an exit for the cancer cells.

Further information

UK

Penny Brohn Cancer Care evidence-based information sheet on imagery (visualization): www.pennybrohncancercare.org/upload/docs/932/imagery.pdf

Cancer Research UK: www.cancerhelp.org.uk/about-cancer/treatment/complementary-alternative/therapies/visualisation

US

Kaiser-Permanente, a US Health Management organization, offers free downloadable visualization exercises for cancer patients: http://members.kaiserpermanente.org/redirects/listen/?kp_shortcut_referrer=kp.org/listen

The Cancer Game site has a stress-relief game for cancer patients in which they can visualize and destroy cancer on a computer screen: www.cancergame.org

Clinical trial on *Relaxation and Visualization Therapy for Breast Cancer Patients* from the **US National Institutes of Health**: http://clinicaltrials.gov/ct2/show/NCT00691119

Examples of visualizations can be found at **Healing Cancer Naturally**: www.healingcancernaturally.com/cancer-healing-visualizations.html

References

Guided Imagery for Self-Healing by Martin Rossman. H.J. Kramer (2000).

Creative Power of Imagery: A Practical Guide to the Workings of Your Mind by Ian Gawler. Michelle Anderson Publishing (2000).

You Can Conquer Cancer by Dr Ian Gawler. Michelle Anderson Publishing (2002).

V is for Vitamins

Vitamins A, C and E – which have antioxidant properties – are covered in 'A is for Antioxidant Vitamins and Minerals', and folic acid (one of the B group of vitamins) has its own section. But we must also consider the importance of vitamin D.

This essential substance is produced in our skin when it is exposed to sunlight, as well as being available in small quantities in eggs, liver and oily fish, and as an additive in margarine and some breakfast cereals. Vitamin D is required for the formation of healthy bones (having too little leads to rickets). Vitamin D and calcium supplements may help reduce bone loss in women who have passed the menopause and in those being treated with breast cancer drugs (especially aromatase inhibitors) that deplete bone by blocking production of oestrogen. But there is also great interest in evidence that vitamin D may reduce the risk of developing certain cancers.

Laboratory work suggests that vitamin D reduces the proliferation of breast cancer cells, and that it encourages malignant cells to 'differentiate' – that is, to become more like their normal counterparts. But the best evidence of benefit comes from studies which relate cancer rates in large groups of people to levels of vitamin D and its metabolites measured in their blood. The data are reasonably consistent in showing that higher vitamin D levels are associated with lower risk of breast and colon cancer. There seems to be no protective effect of vitamin D against certain other tumours such as melanoma, and the evidence relating to reduced risk of prostate and pancreatic cancers is not consistent.

TOP TIP

Vitamin D can cause toxicities and, especially if you have cancer, it would be wise to consult your doctor before taking supplements.

Further information

UK

See **Penny Brohn Cancer Care's** *The Bristol Approach to Supplements: A guide to how to maintain optimal nutrient levels whilst living with cancer* (2010) downloadable from: www.pennybrohncancercare.org/upload/docs/932/pbcc_supplement_guidelines_2010.pdf

Cancer Research UK: www.cancerhelp.org.uk/about-cancer/treatment/
complementary-alternative/about/harm/the-safety-of-vitamins-and-diet-
supplements

US

American Cancer Society on vitamins: www.cancer.org/Treatment/
TreatmentsandSideEffects/ComplementaryandAlternativeMedicine/
HerbsVitaminsandMinerals/index

For **Lewis Gale Hospital's** information on vitamins, go to the website, scroll
down to 'Natural and Alternative Treatments' on the main menu and click
on 'Herbs and Supplements'. Then find 'Vitamins and minerals (general)' in
the A–Z list, or select the particular vitamin that you want to find out about:
www.alleghanyregional.com/healthcontent.asp?page=contentselection/
condensedmainindex

Information from the **Linus Pauling Institute**: http://lpi.oregonstate.edu/
infocenter/vitamins.html

References

'Vitamin D for cancer prevention: Global perspective' by C.F. Garland and colleagues. *Annals of Epidemiology* 2009, volume 19, pages 468–483.

'Vitamin D and cancer incidence in the Harvard cohorts' by Edward Giovannucci. *Annals of Epidemiology* 2009, volume 19, pages 84–88.

W is for Weight

Since living with cancer, every time I go for a treatment or check up, I am immediately escorted to the scales. I ask if I have lost any weight, as the digits escalate in front of me. Weight loss is often a sign of active cancer, but as I write I am heavier than I have ever been. I have been told not to diet and find it incredibly difficult to just eat sensibly.

Sensible eating is of course the key – particularly if you have lost weight due to chemotherapy or radiation treatment. The body has already suffered infiltration of toxic substances, and you do not want to place it under more stress by yet more toxins in fast or junk food. (See also 'D is for Diet and Nutritional Therapy (or Food, Glorious Food)'.)

Having just returned from skiing with my godchildren, I am four pounds heavier. Easy with extremely fattening foods such as cheese fondue – organic cheese melted with a little organic milk and wholemeal bread dunked in. Mmm! Chocolate fondue – chocolate melted with a little hot water and then cut bananas, pineapple or pears in bite-size dunkable shape. Also mmm! Organic pasta is readily available in all shapes and sizes, and you can add a variety of yummy quickly prepared, freshly made sauces.

TOP TIP

The silver lining in the cloud of regaining weight is that you really are allowed to eat a lot of what you fancy – but remember what you fancy may not be good for you. If in doubt, visit a professionally trained dietician or nutritionist.

Further information

UK

Macmillan Cancer Support: www.macmillan.org.uk/Cancerinformation/ Livingwithandaftercancer/Eatingwell/Thebuilding-updiet/Overview.aspx

The Bristol Approach 7 Day Recipe Plan by Elizabeth Butler, Senior Nutritional Therapist, and Anna Ralph, Head Chef, Penny Brohn Cancer Care, accompanies the Bristol Approach to Healthy Eating, a set of guidelines to support the general health and well-being of those with cancer (2010). Downloadable from **Penny Brohn Cancer Care**: www.shopatpennybrohn. com/page51.asp. *The Bristol Approach to Healthy Eating: A Guide on How to Maintain a Healthy Balanced Diet whilst Living with Cancer* (2010) is downloadable from www.pennybrohncancercare.org/page37.asp

US

The **American Cancer Society** offers nutritional guidelines for cancer patients: www.cancer.org/docroot/MBC/MBC_6.asp?sitearea=ETO

US National Cancer Institute information on nutrition in cancer care: www.cancer.gov/cancertopics/pdq/supportivecare/nutrition/Patient/page1

References

Say No to Cancer: The Drug-Free Guide to Preventing and Helping Fight Cancer by Patrick Holford. Piatkus Books (2010).

Nutrition and Cancer State-of-the-Art by Sandra Goodman. Health Research Ltd (2003), available from www.drsgoodman.com/books-goodman.

Healing Foods Cookbook: The Vegan Way to Wellness by Jane Sen. Thorsons (2002).

W is for Wigs

See 'C is for Cold Cap' for how *not* to lose your hair – but if it does happen, this is your opportunity to (1) appear in heavy disguise and see who recognizes you and (2) see if blondes really do have more fun!

But it is the most miserable experience – not just losing your hair but eyelashes and eyebrows. It's very difficult to see the silver lining in that particular dark cloud – even with beautiful hair-free legs. And hair loss makes you a marked woman. A solicitor explained that all was going well at first. She was back at work after the surgery. And then she lost her hair, followed by most of her clients. In this world of tough dealing, they did not want any sign of weakness – such as cancer – to enter the equation. This could have been an error on the part of the clients because cancer may make you more steadfast and more true.

I acknowledged the strong possibility of losing my hair and went and looked at wigs. I was not even remotely tempted by a real hair wig because it is as difficult to manage as any real hair. The look-like-real, feel-like-real but fake hair option was the one for me. Wash with warm soapy water (careful with this if you have a sensitive scalp – so no chemicals), rinse, shake and it falls completely perfectly into its dear little cut. Then leave to dry naturally on its polystyrene head stand. (Some wigs come with a warning not to use any heat such as with hairdryers and tongs. Is this in case they melt?)

Now comes the trick: I chose a wig which was exactly the same colour as my own carefully coloured and highlighted hair, which was at the time longer. I then went to my hairdressers wearing my wig. I was greeted with anger and despair as they jumped to the conclusion that I had had my hair cut elsewhere. At which point I pulled off my wig. So first test passed – at a distance my wig looked like my real hair and even fooled the professionals. Then I produced the headstand, put the wig on it and explained I wanted my own hair cut exactly like it. I left the hairdressers wig in hand – well, handbag.

For the next few weeks I went through all the usual oohs and aahs – from friends, family and acquaintances – that you get when you suddenly change a hairstyle you have had for years. Those who thought I had already lost my hair and pulled were surprised by my reaction – a loud screech! So, when I eventually did lose my hair, on went the wig and there was absolutely no reaction from anyone – with the exception of a very dear friend who knew how nervous and self-conscious I would feel wearing my wig. She arrived for tennis with not a hair out of place. I noticed the new smart cut and how lovely it looked – and it still looked lovely after tennis, but then she took it off! 'There you are,' she said. 'No one knows except you!' She made it so much easier for me, and I hope recounting the tale makes it a whole lot easier for you.

Looking back, it was just a brief moment of time. My hair is lovely now, thicker than ever, as are my eyelashes, and I am sure they are longer!

TOP TIP

Try before you buy.

Further information

UK

Cancer Research UK information on obtaining wigs through the NHS: www.cancerhelp.org.uk/about-cancer/cancer-questions/hair-loss-and-wigs#nhs

Trendco Hair Supplies, Sheridan House, 114/116 Western Road, Hove, East Sussex BN3 1DD. Tel: 01273 774977/777503. Website: www.trendco.co.uk

Hair to Wear, Jacquelyn Collection International, 16 Seymour Court, Cazenove Road, London N16 6AU. Tel: 020 8806 8751. Email: jacqwigsuk@aol.com

Most major department stores have wig departments.

US

American Cancer Society information on hair loss accessories (scroll to bottom of page): www.cancer.org/Cancer/BreastCancer/MoreInformation/breast-prostheses-and-hair-loss-accessories-list

W is for Work

I have struggled with the work/play balance most of my life. With a diagnosis of cancer, I have managed to get something of a balance that did not seem achievable prior to that diagnosis.

First, it is important for your whole being to be happy in your work. To be struggling with difficult, unpleasant people is something to be avoided, in the same way as you avoid all other negatives in life. Work is meant to be enjoyed and to be fulfilling and rewarding. If it is not, then it may be time to make those changes. A diagnosis of cancer is the perfect time for a re-evaluation.

The Equality Act 2010 means that people with cancer (and also HIV and multiple sclerosis) are protected from discrimination at work, in education, in access to goods and services and in buying or renting property. So you cannot be turned down for a promotion simply because you have cancer or have had cancer. It is unlawful for an employer to treat someone with cancer less favourably than someone without cancer, and cancer sufferers cannot be made redundant for reasons relating to their condition – except in extreme circumstances. Employers also have a duty to make reasonable adjustments to their employment practices and premises if these place people with cancer at a substantial disadvantage.

TOP TIP

Work hard, play hard – but don't forget you can do both better if you take some rest.

Y is for Yoga

Yoga is a holistic healing system for creating harmony and balance on all levels: body, mind, heart and spirit. When this balance has been disturbed by serious illness, practising yoga can help in a number of ways to restore it. Yoga encourages the development of our inner resources and qualities: the resilience and stability, the clarity and detachment, the self-awareness, acceptance and trust that enable us to meet the challenge of a life-changing illness and to use it as an opportunity for growth and change. It has proved to be a source of support and spiritual nourishment for many people who are living with cancer. Yoga is not a 'cure' for cancer but it can help to strengthen the immune system and encourage our inner healing forces. It works in various ways.

Yoga exercises, known as *asanas*, or postures, influence our breathing, circulation, digestion and elimination, our mental and emotional balance, our nervous system and energy levels, our physical strength, stability, and flexibility, and the way we hold and use ourselves. They enhance the functioning of all our internal organs and systems. To many people in the Western world, the word 'yoga' suggests the impressive physical contortions made popular by celebrities, but these aren't suitable for most people and they aren't necessary. There are many simple, doable exercises that have particular benefits for people who have cancer, practices that encourage full movement of the joints and improve circulation and the functioning of the vital organs, and also help to speed the removal of toxic waste from the body, thus enhancing energy flow. Such simple practices are suitable for everyone, of any age. You don't need to stand on your head or tie yourself in knots.

Breathing exercises (see also 'B is for Breath and Breathing') help to develop the efficient breathing habits that are such an important aspect of general health. On the physical level, the simple breathing and stretching exercises of yoga improve the strength, elasticity and efficiency of the breathing muscles. They also release tension, anxiety and stress, and replenish energy.

Steady, rhythmic breathing calms the sympathetic nervous system (the part of the nervous system that triggers the 'fight or flight' response) and activates the parasympathetic nervous system (the part that gives the body and mind the message that all is well). Healthy breathing habits restore emotional balance and tranquillity, and just a few minutes' daily practice is calming, uplifting and revitalizing.

Relaxation is an especially vital element in healing, because it helps to undo the tension and stress that are so detrimental to the immune system. Relaxation techniques calm the nerves, lower heart rate and blood pressure, dissolve physical and mental tension, and improve concentration and sleep. Regularly practised, they alleviate the stress and anxiety that depress immune function. Through relaxation, we actively cooperate with our immune system and encourage our inner healing forces. We learn to let go and experience inner stillness and peace.

Meditation allows our thoughts and emotions to surface so that we can look at them. The simple meditation practice of breath awareness develops the mental focus, detachment and clarity that help us to look at the reality of our situation, to see things as they are. Then we can acknowledge and accept them, work with them and move forward with our lives. The emotions that accompany a cancer diagnosis – shock, fear, anger and grief among them – are powerful and difficult to bear, and we may be tempted to bury them. But while burying our emotions blocks our energy and increases stress, acknowledging and accepting them liberates energy and reduces stress. Meditation allows repressed emotions to surface and become integrated into consciousness, where they lose their power over us, and this develops the clarity that empowers us to meet the challenges of cancer diagnosis and treatment. Through meditation we are helped to look at the realities of the illness, so that we can move from fear, anger and despair to acceptance and purposeful living. Meditation is therapeutic and healing in the fullest sense of the word.

All these aspects of yoga – movement, breathing, relaxation and meditation – work together holistically to support the healing process and restore balance and harmony when one is dealing with a life-changing illness.

Further information

UK

Julie Friedeberger, 16 Coleraine Road, Blackheath, London SE3 7PQ. Email: juliefried@clara.co.uk. Julie Friedeberger has been practising and teaching yoga for almost 40 years. Her experience of breast cancer in 1993 left her with a deeper trust in the effectiveness of simple yoga practices, and her focus since then has been on the healing potential of yoga.

Cancer Research UK: www.cancerhelp.org.uk/about-cancer/treatment/complementary-alternative/therapies/yoga

Yoga Biomedical Trust: www.yogatherapy.org

The British Wheel of Yoga, 25 Jermyn Street, Sleaford, Lincolnshire NG34 7RU. Tel: 01529 306851. Email: office@bwy.org.uk. Website: www.bwy.org.uk

US

American Cancer Society: www.cancer.org/Treatment/Treatmentsand SideEffects/ComplementaryandAlternativeMedicine/MindBodyandSpirit/yoga

Moffit Cancer Center: www.moffitt.org/CCJRoot/v12n3/pdf/165.pdf

National Center for Complementary and Alternative Medicine: http://nccam.nih.gov/health/yoga/introduction.htm

References

'Effect of YOCAS yoga on sleep, fatigue and quality of life: A randomized controlled trial among 410 cancer survivors' by K.M. Mustian and colleagues. *Journal of Clinical Oncology* 2010, volume 28, abstract 9013 (paper presented at the 2010 annual meeting of the American Society for Clinical Oncology).

'Effects of yoga versus walking on mood, anxiety and brain GABA levels: A randomized, controlled study' by Chris Streeter and colleagues. *Journal of Alternative and Complementary Medicine* 2010, volume 16, pages 1145–1152.

A Visible Wound: A Healing Journey through Breast Cancer by Julie Friedeberger. New Age Books (2004).

The Healing Power of Yoga: for Health, Well-Being and Inner Peace by Julie Friedeberger. New Age Books (2004).

Breathe and Relax: A Way to Healing CD by Julie Friedeberger (see contact details above).

Experience Yoga Nidra: Guided Deep Relaxation (CD) by Swami Janakananda Saraswati. Scandinavian Yoga and Meditation School (1996).

Z is for Zulu Warrior – the Bravest and Finest of African Warriors

U *you can do this*

L *look, listen and learn*

U *you are here – stay in the moment*

'Zulu Warrior' represents the power deep within oneself to fight cancer. It is so important for you and those around you to keep a positive attitude whilst battling against this disease. Be like the Zulu Warrior: arm yourself for battle, with knowledge and by keeping fit, both mentally and physically.

The Zulu Warrior uses 'warpaint' – you can do the same. Take the time to look after your skin, apply a little warpaint of your own, and you will look and feel better for it. Your confidence and self-esteem will benefit. (See 'B is for Beauty'.)

Look, listen and learn: use the power of knowledge to work with your medical team towards recovery. There are so many reasons to be positive and full of hope.

Let the Zulu Warrior in us fight this illness with all the passion and strength we possess. *I know you can overcome the odds. Be ready to do battle and to WIN.*

TOP TIP

Take whatever exercise you feel able to, whether it is a gentle stroll in the park or a game of tennis with friends. Engage in something that gives you pleasure as well as enhancing your overall fitness. That way you will positively look forward to it and continue. Prepare your body for the fight with rest, yes, but also by keeping fit and eating well.

Further information
Reference

Zulu Rising: The Epic Story of iSandlwana and Rorke's Drift by Ian Knight. Macmillan (2010).

Useful Organizations and Websites

United Kingdom

Penny Brohn Cancer Care
Penny Brohn Cancer Care, Chapel Pill Lane, Pill, Bristol BS20 0HH
Freephone: 0845 123 2310, 9.30 a.m. to 5 p.m. Monday to Friday
www.pennybrohncancercare.org

Cancer Research UK
Freephone: 0808 800 40 40, 9 a.m. to 5 p.m. Monday to Friday
www.cancerhelp.org.uk

Macmillan Cancer Support
Freephone: 0808 808 0000
www.macmillan.org.uk
Cancer support specialists (Cancerbackup has now merged with Macmillan).

Breakthrough Breast Cancer
Freephone: 08080 100 200
www.breakthrough.org.uk

Breast Cancer Campaign
Tel: 020 7749 4114
www.breastcancercampaign.org

Marie Curie Cancer Care
Helpline: 0800 716 146, 9 a.m. to 5.30 p.m. Monday to Friday
www.maricurie.org.uk

NHS Choices
www.nhs.uk

NHS Directory of Complementary and Alternative Practitioners
www.nhsdirectory.org

NHS Evidence – Complementary and alternative medicine (CAM)
www.library.nhs.uk/CAM

Research Council for Complementary Medicine
The Royal London Hospital for Integrated Medicine, 60 Great Ormond
Street, London, WC1 3HR
www.rccm.org.uk

Institute for Complementary and Natural Medicine
Can-Mazzanine, 32–36 Loman Street, London SE1 0EH
Tel: 020 7922 7980
www.i-c-m.org.uk

British Complementary Medicine Association
PO Box 5122, Bournemouth BH8 0WG
Tel: 0845 345 5977
www.bcma.co.uk

Cancernet-UK
www.cancernet.co.uk

United States

United States National Cancer Institute
www.cancer.gov
Provides authoritative information on a wide range of cancers and their
treatment, including complementary and alternative approaches. Also
has sections on coping with cancer and cancer prevention, and provides
factsheets.

American Cancer Society
www.cancer.org

American Society of Clinical Oncology
www.cancer.net/portal/site/patient
Site for patients.

National Coalition for Cancer Survivorship (NCCS)
www.canceradvocacy.org

National Comprehensive Cancer Network
www.nccn.com
Patient information site.

Patient Resource Cancer Guide
http://patientresource.net
Has an extensive list of resources for cancer patients.

Cancer Support Community
www.thewellnesscommunity.org

Gilda's Club
www.gildasclub.org/ourclubhouses.asp
Offers a variety of free support services to cancer patients including educational programmes, cancer-specific support groups, Tai Chi, yoga, nutrition education, and programmes for children.

ConsumerLab.com
www.consumerlab.com
This organization's mission is 'to identify the best quality health and nutritional products by independent testing'. It was founded by an MD and a former FDA natural products chemist as an independent testing service for herb and dietary supplement content and issues of contamination and safety. They were the first to bring to widespread attention the fact that some herbal products can contain toxic levels of cadmium, mercury and even uranium – depending on where the plant is grown. There is a small fee to receive their newsletter and have online access to their reviews.

Australia

Cancer Council Australia
Helpline: 13 11 20
www.cancer.org.au

Australian Cancer Research Foundation
Tel: 02 9223 7833
www.acrf.com.au
Email: info@acrf.com.au

McGrath Foundation
PO Box 4, Northbridge, NSW 2063
Tel: (02) 8962 6100
www.mcgrathfoundation.com.au
A breast cancer charity.

CanTeen
Freephone: 1800 226 833
www.canteen.org.au
For young people living with cancer.

Health Direct Australia
www.healthinsite.gov.au/topics/Complementary_and_Alternative_
Therapies

Australia Integrative Medicine Association
www.aima.net.au

Canada

Canadian Cancer Society
www.cancer.ca

Marilyn Van Stone Cancer Care Foundation
www.mvsfoundation.org
Email: info@mvsfoundation.org

Canadian Breast Cancer Foundation
Freephone: 1 (800) 387-9816
www.cbcf.org

Natural Healthcare Canada
http://naturalhealthcare.ca

Canadian Wellness Directory of Alternative Medicine Professionals
www.canadianwellness.com/alternative/alternative_associations.asp

Worldwide

Pubmed
Key this word into a search engine and you have access to 19 million articles
in scholarly journals from throughout the world. Generally, you will find
only a summary (abstract) of these papers but some offer links that will take
you without charge to the full text.

ClinicalTrials.gov
www.clinicaltrials.gov
This US-based website has information on 90,000 clinical trials being
conducted in more than 150 countries. Many are recruiting patients in the
UK, and some may be relevant to you.

Sources of Nutritional Supplements

United Kingdom

The following companies produce/stock good-quality supplements that are widely available in the United Kingdom.

Solgar

Available in most independent health food stores or visit www.solgar-vitamins.co.uk. Tel: 01442 890 355

Biocare

An extensive range of nutritional and herbal supplements, including daily 'packs', ideal for travelling or when away from home. Their products are stocked by most good health-food shops or visit www.biocare.co.uk. Tel: 0121 433 3727

Totally Nourish

An e-health shop stocking many good-quality health products, including home-test kits and supplements. Visit www.totallynourish.com. Tel: 0800 085 7749 (freephone within the UK)

Vitabiotics

An extensive range of nutritional products made to the highest pharmaceutical standards available from Boots, Waitrose, Holland & Barrett and online at www.vitabiotics.com. Tel: 020 8955 2600

The Nutri Centre, London

Prince Charles opened the centre in 1988 and today it is the UK's leading supplier of nutritional products stocking a vast range of vitamins, herbs and homeopathic medicines. The centre offers same-day dispatch for phone or email orders and also has in-house nutritional consultants, happy to give advice. Tel (for mail order and general enquiries): 0845 602 6744. Tel (for nutritionists): 020 7436 5122. Website: www.nutricentre.com

Penny Brohn Cancer Care (formerly Bristol Cancer Help Centre)
A wide range of nutritional and herbal supplements including their Bristol Approach Supplement Packs. Stockists of Biocare and other leading brands. Freephone: 0845 123 23 10, 9.30 a.m. to 5 p.m. weekdays. Website: www.pennybrohncancercare.org

Jan De Vries Healthcare
Jan De Vries Healthcare has an online health store stocking supplements and homeopathic and herbal remedies. The store stocks a range of brands including Biocare, A Vogel and Jan De Vries products.

United States

In the United States, supplements are not regulated by the Food and Drug Administration and often vary in quality and purity. However, products frequently carry seals to indicate that they have been tested or meet basic standards.

If a product carries the ConsumerLab.com quality seal or is listed on their website as having passed their random independent testing programme, you can be assured the supplement is high-quality and should perform as expected.

The USP or NSF seal means that the producer claims the product meets the relevant US Pharmacopoeia or National Formulary standards. Among other things, these standards cover potency, minimum dosage and purity from contamination.

The National Nutritional Food Association's (NNFA) GMP seal indicates the manufacturer has passed a comprehensive, independent inspection of its manufacturing process. This gives solid assurance of a well-made product but says nothing about the manufacturer's choice of ingredients and potency levels.

A product that carries the BioFIT trademark has passed 'biological assay' testing, which means that it displays biochemical activity that is consistent with having the corresponding effect in the human body.

The Supplement Watch Seal: SupplementWatch.com uses a subjective, 100-point system for rating brands. Up to 20 points are awarded for each of five categories: health claims, scientific theory, scientific research, safety and side effects, and value (relative cost).

ConsumerLab lists the vendors given below as reputable and as carrying some of the products they have tested. Not all products offered by these vendors have been tested for quality by ConsumerLab. Prices at some of these suppliers may be less than in drug and health food stores.

- Swansonvitamins.com
- iHerb.com
- VitaminLife.com
- LuckyVitamin.com
- Puritan's Pride: www.puritan.com
- Vitacost.com
- eVitamins.com

INDEX